Bioethics
Across the Life Span

Bioethics Across the Life Span

EDITED BY MARILYN E. COORS

THE NATIONAL CATHOLIC BIOETHICS CENTER

Philadelphia

Cover design by Nicholas Furton
ISBN 978-0-935372-67-0

Unless otherwise noted, quotations from Scripture are from the
Revised Standard Version, Catholic Edition, prepared by the Catholic
Biblical Association of Great Britain © 1965, 1966 National
Council of the Churches of Christ in the United States of America;
quotations from Church documents are from the Vatican English
translation, published online at www.vatican.va © Libreria Editrice
Vaticana; and quotations from the Catechism are from the *Catechism
of the Catholic Church*, 2nd ed. © 1994, 1997 United States Catholic
Conference, Inc. / Libreria Editrice Vaticana.

Library of Congress Cataloging-in-Publication Data

Bioethics across the life span / edited by Marilyn E. Coors.
   p. ; cm.
  Includes bibliographical references.
  ISBN 978-0-935372-67-0 (alk. paper)
  I. Coors, Marilyn E., 1947- , editor. II. National Catholic Bioethics
Center, issuing body.
  [DNLM: 1. Bioethical Issues. 2. Catholicism. 3. Religion and Medi-
cine. WB 60]
  R725.56
  241'.642--dc23

                   2015027209

To Janet, Therese, and Sister Prudence, who persistently encouraged me to bring this book to print.

Contents

PREFACE

Called to be standard bearers for human dignity, Catholics should openly affirm the truth. In his address to the students of the Jesuit schools of Italy and Albania on June 7, 2013, Pope Francis summoned his flock to be free and courageous in the defense of dignity, especially as contemporary culture is frequently enchanted with consumerism and blinded to the deeper meaning of life:

> First of all: be free people! ... Freedom means being able to think about what we do, being able to assess what is good and what is bad, these are the types of conduct that lead to development. ... Always being free to choose goodness is demanding but it will make you into people with a backbone who can face life, people with courage.

Be free to make informed, reasoned, and bold assessments that serve the greatest good for humankind—let it always be a yes to protect human life, even life that is heavily burdened.

Preface

Science and technology have made possible things that were unthinkable to previous generations—designer babies, organ transplantation, mechanical ventilation—some that threaten and others that promote the dignity of human beings. When ethical questions arise, Catholics turn to an accurate moral compass to guide them through these complex matters—the teaching of the Church. Every chapter in this book demonstrates that reality. Whether considering in vitro fertilization or removing life support from a loved one, the Church provides teachings that lead the faithful to a moral response of love. Thus, the purpose of this book is to provide a source in accordance with Pope Francis's call "to raise awareness and form the lay faithful, in whatever state, especially those engaged in the field of politics, so that they may think in accord with the Gospel and the Social Doctrine of the Church and act consistently" (address of Pope Francis to a delegation from the *Dignitatis Humanae* Institute, December 7, 2013).

Unlike many secular bioethicists who question its meaning and usefulness, Catholic teaching clearly articulates dignity as the overarching standard by which to assess the morality of actions. Because each person is created in the image of God, the Church describes human dignity as the inviolable value of every human life. (See, for example, Gen. 1:26–27, as well as the *Catechism*, n. 1700, and *Gaudium et spes*, n. 26). For this reason, life is sacred from the moment of conception and through all subsequent stages to natural death. In his December 7, 2013, address to members of the *Dignitatis Humanae* Institute, an international organization that promotes human dignity, Pope Francis cautioned the attendees regarding a "false model" of humanity:

> Unfortunately, in our own time, one so rich in achievements and hopes, there are many powers and forces that end up producing a culture of waste; and this tends to become the common mentality. ... The victims of this culture are precisely the weakest and most fragile human beings—the unborn, the poorest, the sick and elderly, the seriously handicapped, et al.—who are in danger of being "thrown away," expelled by a system that must be efficient at all costs.

In this complex and distracted culture, human dignity provides the foundation upon which to make bioethical judgments regarding the fundamental questions of human existence.

Overview

This book discusses the nature of bioethics, key topics that fall into this category, their implications for our everyday lives, and their ramifications to the larger family of humankind. The authors include interdisciplinary voices from well-known bioethicists and theologians on current issues, provide instruction on topics on which the Church has ruled, and leave open for further study those questions in bioethics about which the Church has not decided. The audience for this work includes educators and students in bioethics, health professionals, hospital administrators and staff, and readers with an interest in bioethics with either little or extensive background on the subject. The topics were chosen through interviews that asked Catholics to identify bioethical questions that were important in their lives and about which they wanted more information.

The work begins with an introduction to bioethics by Erica Laethem, regional director of ethics at OSF Health Care in Rockford, Illinois. She describes the origins of bioethics, explains why it is interdisciplinary, and discusses the morality of human action. Laethem uses pertinent cases and examples from everyday life to illustrate important ethical concepts, including human action and moral precepts.

In chapter 2, John Haas, who serves on the governing council of the Pontifical Academy of Life and is president of The National Catholic Bioethics Center in Philadelphia, provides a well-informed and sensitive approach to assisted reproductive technologies. He explains the science and discusses the morality of various means of overcoming infertility. The Church does not reject any means of overcoming infertility merely because it is artificial—a common misconception. Thus, Haas provides a "rule of thumb" to assist Catholics in analyzing and deciding for themselves if a given technological intervention is moral or immoral according to Church teaching.

In chapter 3, Edward Furton, an ethicist and the director of publications at The National Catholic

Bioethics Center, tackles a topic about which there is some controversy among well-meaning Catholics: vaccines, their link to cell lines obtained from aborted fetuses, and the real-world ramifications. Since some vaccines currently in use have their origin in cell lines produced from fetal tissue aborted in the distant past, Furton walks the reader through a detailed analysis of what constitutes cooperation in an immoral action and recommends a way forward. Chapter 3 also includes answers to frequently asked questions about vaccines.

The remainder of the work focuses on bioethical questions related to medical procedures and genetics in health care. Science and ethics are intertwined in these chapters, because good facts are critical to good ethics. Chapter 4 discusses the science and morality of rape protocols and emergency contraception, another topic that engenders discussion among Catholics. The reasons for the debate include the uncertainty regarding the action of the protocol drugs, and the potential immorality of the treatment depending on the timing in the victim's cycle, which is sometimes difficult to measure. Haas, the author of chapter 4, uses the virtue of prudence to address the role of certitude in making moral decisions in health care, which takes into account the ambiguities in knowledge arising from human limitations and the various circumstances that surround any action.

In chapter 5, Furton addresses the sometimes misunderstood topic of organ donation from both living and deceased donors. He explains the two methods of determining death prior to organ donation: the traditional cardio-pulmonary method and the newer neurological or brain death methods, especially in relation to Pope St. John Paul II's Address to the 18th International Congress on Transplants in August 2000. The real life examples presented by Furton provide clear guidance in understanding the moral and ethical issues involved in organ donation as a gift of life.

Chapters 6 and 7 are authored by Marilyn Coors, who is an associate professor of bioethics and genetics at the University of Colorado Anschutz Medical Campus. Chapter 6 takes the topic of adult, embryonic, and induced pluripotent stem cells as an example of a bioethical issue that embroils morality, science, power, and politics in contentious public debate. The author relies on the standards articulated in the 2008 Congregation for the Doctrine of the Faith instruction *Dignitas personae* to explore how embryonic stem cell research devalues human life. She examines the connection between the procurement of human eggs for embryonic stem cell research and the exploitation of women as illustrated in the public press. Chapter 7 considers the scientific and moral aspects of genetic screening and testing that Catholics encounter through medical efforts to diagnose the cause of disease or disability affecting themselves or their families. The chapter also discusses current and futuristic applications of genetic engineering and outlines the timeless criteria of human dignity that must be met for genetic interventions to be moral.

The Most Reverend José Gomez, Archbishop of Los Angeles, begins chapter 8 with a description of the Christian meaning of death and then explores the morality of end-of-life issues, including euthanasia, the persistent vegetative state, and rational limits to medical treatment. The Archbishop employs the concept of "therapeutic tyranny" to consider the meaning of suffering and the notion of authentic mercy in a medical context. He concludes the chapter and the book by encouraging Catholics to build a "culture of life" that cultivates and defends human dignity in all its stages and recovers culture's most essential element, which is a human being's relationship with God.

Catholics must think through these current bioethical topics with the mind of the Church. Often, Catholics get their news the way the rest of the world does—from television, print media, and the internet. When good-hearted but often under-informed Catholics hear about the Church's opposition or endorsement of some scientific research, they sometimes express frustration and confusion, in part, because they do not understand the moral reasoning that undergirds the position. The aim of this book is to cut through the confusion and invite Catholics to understand the meaning of bioethics within Catholic moral teaching.

MARILYN E. COORS

Bioethics
Across the Life Span

I

WHY BOTHER WITH BIOETHICS?

Erica Laethem

Few of us will escape this life without facing at least one bioethical question. Though the field of bioethics may seem like the esoteric musings of academics, in reality it is quite practical.

For some, the question will arise in a pediatrician's office, when the physician recommends a series of vaccinations for a child. You try to keep abreast of the best medical advice for your children, and perhaps you are supportive of vaccinations in general, but have heard that some vaccinations may contain components that were obtained using immoral means. And if they did, would it be okay to use these vaccines if there were no other effective ways of preventing the illnesses? What are the risks? What are the benefits? Is it worth it? If you give your consent for inoculation, does it mean that you condone the immoral origins of the vaccines, or are there ways to use them morally?

For others, the question will arise around the dinner table, when aging parents tell the family that they have been talking to their doctors about advance care planning. They are creating advance directives and want to talk with you about their health care preferences. Your mother tells you that in light of her progressing dementia, she does not want to be resuscitated, and she thinks that a feeding tube is more than she could ever handle—and besides, she says, her doctor told her that it is not recommended for patients with dementia. She says that she wants to die at home, to be in a familiar environment surrounded by the loving care of her family. She asks you to serve as her durable-power-of-attorney-for-health-care agent, to make health-care decisions on her behalf in the event that she is not able to speak for herself. She leans forward, takes your hand in hers, and says that she hopes that you will consider hospice if she has less than six months to live. It all seems very reasonable, but are there other questions that you should ask or things that you should know before her illness gets to that point?

For some of us, the question will arise at the office, when a colleague tells us that after a long struggle with infertility, she and her husband have met a gifted physician, a reproductive endocrinologist, who has shown them photos of the beautiful families he has helped create and has offered to do the same for them. With hope in her eyes, she speaks about the range of interventions her physician has presented and asks what you think she should do.

For others still, the question will arise in your professional work in health care, when you are asked to assist in an organ donation, or to provide post-traumatic care for a victim of sexual assault, or to help a devastated and divided family decide whether to withdraw life-sustaining treatment and focus exclusively on providing comfort-care measures for a loved one. How do we approach these things with compassion and integrity?

Yes, few of us will escape this life without facing bioethical questions. Often, though not always, these questions arise at times in our lives, or the lives of our friends, family members, coworkers, or patients, that are naturally stressful and emotionally draining, times when it is difficult to think through all the possibilities and implications in a thoughtful and thorough way. Sometimes decisions have to be made quickly, and responses need to be given seemingly on the spot; to do so well, it helps to have thought through some of these questions before we are in the throes of crisis.

The purpose of bioethics is to help us make good decisions and, in particular, good decisions in the fields of medicine and science. In the Catholic Tradition, the ultimate purpose of morality is to help us love, and this has implications for bioethics.

What Is Bioethics?

The word "ethics" comes from the Greek *ethos*, meaning custom, a habitual way of acting, or more simply, character. The Latin words *mos* and *mosis,* from which the English words *mores* and *morals* are derived, have the same meaning. Ethics is a philosophical science, meaning that its method is rational argument. Moral theology, on the other hand, is a theological science, where the starting point is faith and the method is reflection on divine revelation— the Sacred Scriptures and Apostolic Tradition. In the Catholic moral tradition, the discipline of bioethics emerged within the broader fields of ethics and moral theology.

Bioethics is a systematic way of addressing ethical questions that arise in medicine and science. Its focus is the study of morally relevant human action. Its methodology, depending on the approach, involves rational thought (philosophy) or faith seeking understanding (theology), or both.

Bioethics is a practical science, as opposed to a purely speculative one. It involves the science as well as the art of applying abstract concepts and principles to concrete situations. To do this art well, one needs knowledge of the relevant ethical principles, astute reasoning skills, and an understanding of the reality that is being assessed. To assess that reality, one needs to start with the facts of the situation.

Gathering the facts generally involves fields of study other than theology or ethics. The Church's magisterium, or official teaching office, makes pronouncements only on matters of faith and morals, not on science. In *Dignitas personae*, the Congregation for the Doctrine of the Faith describes this role: "The Church, by expressing an ethical judgment on some developments of recent medical research concerning man and his beginnings, does not intervene in the area proper to medical science itself, but rather calls everyone to ethical and social responsibility for their actions. ... The intervention of the Magisterium falls within its mission of contributing to the formation of conscience, by authentically teaching the truth which is Christ and at the same time by declaring and confirming authoritatively the principles of the moral order which spring from human nature itself." [1]

Assessing the facts of the situation will usually involve dialogue and collaboration with professionals in medicine, science, law, spiritual care, and others. Input from other fields is necessary to the work of bioethics, since it is impossible to provide a competent bioethical analysis without an adequate grasp of the facts to be analyzed. By its very nature, bioethics is interdisciplinary.

Bioethics approached from a Catholic perspective is part of the mosaic of Catholic Tradition, and it is therefore best understood and carried out in reference to Catholic Tradition as a whole. Discussion of particular bioethical norms and analyses is most properly set in a holistic understanding of the world, salvation, and our place in it—in the dynamism of sin and grace. This helps prevent those of us involved in the work of bioethics, whether as bioethicists or as people making bioethical decisions, from becoming so focused on our detailed analyses that we lose sight of our ultimate purpose, which is to love and to help others to do what is loving.

Any attempt to summarize the rich two-thousand-year tradition of Catholicism, with its Jewish roots that stretch beyond that, will inevitably be inadequate. But because bioethics is most properly understood in reference to the Tradition as a whole, I would like to spend a short time discussing four aspects of Catholic Tradition that help shape our study of bioethics.

The first is *Catholic social teaching*. Foundational to Catholic social teaching is the concept of human dignity, that inherent worthiness of the person that demands respect. All the other principles of Catholic social teaching—respect for human life, life in society, human rights and responsibilities, a preferential option for the poor, the dignity of work and rights of workers, solidarity in pursuit of justice and peace, and stewardship for creation—find their roots in the affirmation of human dignity.

The second is *Christian anthropology*, the study of the human person, which speaks to the sources of human dignity. The Sacred Scriptures reveal that the human person is created "in the image and likeness" of God and is called to life that far exceeds the dimensions of earthly existence, because it consists in sharing in the very life of the Trinity, a life of total self-giving love.[2] The life, death, and resurrection of Jesus further reveal God's love for humanity and shed light on the incomparable value of every person.[3] Human dignity implies worthiness of respect that does not depend on someone's net worth, accumulated degrees, or social prestige; it does not consider what tasks a person can perform or how "useful" he or she is to society; it does not fluctuate with age, health, or beauty, and it does not hinge on intellectual abilities, physical aptitudes, or any other subjective factor. It is a worthiness that comes simply with being a person.

The Congregation for the Doctrine of the Faith describes this inestimable dignity:

> By virtue of the simple fact of existing, every human being must be fully respected. ... At every stage of his existence, man, created in the image and likeness of God, reflects "the face of his Only-begotten Son." ... This boundless and almost incomprehensible love of God for the human being reveals the degree to which the human person deserves to be loved in himself, independently of any other consideration—intelligence, beauty,

health, youth, integrity, and so forth. In short, human life is always a good, for it "is a manifestation of God in the world, a sign of his presence, a trace of his glory."[4]

The great Christian writer C. S. Lewis suggested that "next to the Blessed Sacrament itself, your neighbour is the holiest object presented to your senses."[5] Bioethics approached from a Catholic perspective involves a posture of reverence and respect toward each person, recognizing that each is valued and worthy of love.

A third aspect that shapes bioethics approached from a Catholic perspective is *the natural law tradition*. In the Catholic Tradition, faith and reason are not seen as mutually exclusive but rather as mutually enriching and complementary. Pope St. John Paul II described the relationship, saying that "faith and reason are like two wings on which the human spirit rises to the contemplation of truth."[6] For the Catholic, reason is not something to fear or distrust, but something to affirm and embrace while recognizing its limitations. Further, as Catholics we do not believe that we are the only ones capable of knowing what is good or doing it; to the contrary, we believe that those who do not share our faith still have a certain original moral sense, an innate sense of good and evil, right and wrong. This is called the natural law.

The natural law is what St. Paul spoke about in his Letter to the Romans: "When Gentiles who have not the law do by nature what the law requires, they are a law to themselves, even though they do not have the law. They show that what the law requires is written on their hearts, while their conscience also bears witness and their conflicting thoughts accuse or perhaps excuse them on that day when … God judges the secrets of men by Christ Jesus" (Rom. 2:14–16). "Natural" means in accord with our nature as human beings. The *Catechism of the Catholic Church* explains, "This law is called 'natural,' not in reference to the nature of irrational beings, but because reason which decrees it properly belongs to human nature" (n. 1955).

This is relevant to our discussion of bioethics. One need not be Catholic to share values common to the Catholic Tradition, to affirm its principles, or to reach similar conclusions about bioethical issues. As one Jewish physician and ethics committee chair remarked to me about Catholic teaching regarding nutrition and hydration, "This doesn't strike me as Catholic. It just strikes me as reasonable." Such is evidence of the natural law. One does not have to be a follower of Christ to share these values or affirm these principles.

The natural law tradition influences the Catholic approach to bioethics. Not all Catholic bioethicists will begin an analysis with the Scriptures or with a document of the magisterium; some might start with general ethical principles that all can appreciate. They might not use parochial language, but may opt instead for terms that are more common to the culture. This need not give rise to concern; it is, in fact, a valid way to come to know truth about things and to dialogue with people from a variety of backgrounds. Similarly, one need not immediately dismiss the writings of those who are not approaching bioethics from a uniquely Catholic perspective. Without minimizing the importance of discerning what one accepts, Catholic Tradition affirms that truths can be known through reason and, therefore, that ethicists from other faith traditions and even secular writers can offer useful insights. A Catholic approach to bioethics is one that sees faith and reason as capable of working harmoniously together.

The fourth aspect of Catholic teaching that helps set the context for bioethics is the Gospel message of the love and mercy that God extends to us by becoming man, by dying for our sins, and by being resurrected to redeem our humanity and to invite us to deeper friendship with God. This is a central message of the Church, and as such it influences the way that we approach bioethical discussion. Pope Francis, in an often-quoted but sometimes misunderstood interview, speaks of God's healing love and the good news of salvation as the central truths of the Church's message:

> I see clearly that the thing the Church needs most today is the ability to heal wounds and to warm the hearts of the faithful; it needs nearness, proximity. I see the church as a field hospital after battle. It is

useless to ask a seriously injured person if he has high cholesterol and about the level of his blood sugars! You have to heal his wounds. Then we can talk about everything else. Heal the wounds, heal the wounds. And you have to start from the ground up.

The Church sometimes has locked itself up in small things, in small-minded rules. The most important thing is the first proclamation: Jesus Christ has saved you.[7]

In other words, the rules are not the starting point, and they are not even the ending point. The Church's message begins with the good news of salvation, and ultimately aims at bringing others to encounter the love of God so that a personal relationship can form. Norms, including moral norms, are neither the beginning nor the end, but a means. They offer a way of expressing our love for God and for our neighbor, and a way to live happily, in accord with the way God has made us.

Since bioethics in particular involves the application of norms and guidelines, it is important to see these guidelines in light of their purpose, which is to help us love; otherwise, we risk getting caught up in the "small-minded rules" that Pope Francis warns about. Behind every ethical norm, there is a great good to be protected and promoted. Behind every no is a bigger yes to the dignity and inalienable value of the person.[8] Negative moral precepts ("Thou shall not …") protect us from stooping beneath our dignity and from doing something that is contrary to love of God and love of neighbor. Mindfulness of the whole of the Gospel and our ultimate invitation to be loved and to love in return helps us not focus so myopically on the rules that we forget why they are there.

These four aspects of Catholic Tradition—Catholic social teaching and its emphasis on human dignity; Christian anthropology, which offers an explanation for the source of human dignity; the natural law tradition, which affirms the compatibility of faith and reason; and the Gospel message of salvation, which puts into perspective how the work of bioethics fits into the Church's broader mission—should be kept in mind as we discuss some of the details of bioethical analysis.

Sources of Morality in Human Action and Implications of Human Dignity

Respect for human dignity has real implications. Recognizing that the human person is a union of body and soul, respecting the dignity of the person, implies respecting the dignity of the body as well as the spiritual dimension of the person.[9] Bodily life provides the foundation for all other human values, such as freedom and relationships. In his apostolic exhortation on the vocation and the mission of the lay faithful in the Church and the world, John Paul II spoke of the right to life as a fundamental and inviolable human right: "The common outcry, which is justly made on behalf of human rights—for example, the right to health, to home, to work, to family, to culture—is false and illusory if the right to life, the most basic and fundamental right and the condition for all other personal rights, is not defended with maximum determination."[10] It goes without saying that if a person is deprived of life, all other values are irrelevant.

At the same time, respecting the dignity of the person also implies respecting the spiritual interiority of the person. Catholic Tradition holds in high esteem the moral conscience, and encourages its moral formation. The responsibility to follow one's conscience is discussed in the Second Vatican Council document *Gaudium et spes*:

> In the depths of his conscience, man detects a law which he does not impose upon himself, but which holds him to obedience. Always summoning him to love good and avoid evil, the voice of conscience when necessary speaks to his heart: do this, shun that. For man has in his heart a law written by God; to obey it is the very dignity of man; according to which he will be judged. Conscience is the most secret core and sanctuary of a man. There he is alone with God, Whose voice echoes in his depths.[11]

Human dignity is also the foundation for the personalistic norm, the ethical principle that the human person should always be treated as an end in himself or herself and should never be reduced to a mere means. When applied to biotechnology and medicine, the personalistic norm demands that science and technology must be at the service of the person, and not vice versa.

Conditions for Human Action

But how can one tell whether a particular action is in accord with human dignity? At what point does an action become unworthy of human pursuit? How do circumstances factor into this discussion? Furthermore, are all actions morally relevant, or are there some that are not considered in ethics at all?

First, let us define what is meant by the phrase "human action." There is something particular about those actions that human beings freely and consciously carry out that give them an ethical character. Actions that human beings perform can be grouped into two categories: actions of a human being (*actus hominis*) and specifically human actions (*actus humanus*). Actions of a human being are actions that express those aspects of our nature that we share with other living beings. Our hearts beat, our eyes blink, and we instinctively recoil when we touch a burning stove. These activities, which ethicist Joseph de Finance calls "instinctive, thoughtless movements, mannerisms, reflex actions," do not fall under the lens of ethics.[12] Human actions (*actus humanus*), on the other hand, proceed precisely from those faculties that are specific to human beings—namely, reason and will. These actions are rational, free, conscious, and deliberate.[13] Ethics deals with these kinds of actions. For an action to be truly human, the acting person (the moral agent) must be fully present to himself or herself, must fully know what he or she is choosing to do, and must act freely and voluntarily.

The distinction between acts of a human being and human actions has decisive implications for bioethical analysis. It sheds light on the moral difference between allowing a person with end-stage pancreatic cancer to die comfortably without the burdens of artificial life support and intentionally causing the death of another person through chemical euthanasia, and on the moral difference between recognizing the death of an embryo through spontaneous miscarriage and procuring the death of an embryo through embryo-destructive stem cell research. Only human actions—those freely chosen—are the subject of ethical scrutiny.

Since we do not have access to a person's interior life, we cannot fully know whether a person is acting with full freedom and knowledge. Often people who do what is wrong do not know it is wrong, or they act out of fear or anger or under a constraint that makes the action less "theirs." A person is fully responsible only for actions that are freely and consciously chosen.

Although freedom is a necessary condition for human action, the mere presence of freedom cannot determine whether the action is good or not. Not all actions that are carried out freely are necessarily good. What we choose is important in ethics. I may choose many things freely and voluntarily: I may choose to set up a clinic that offers care for the poor and vulnerable, or I may choose to set up a clinic that deliberately excludes those who lack resources. These are not morally equivalent decisions. We are called to pursue the good, but how can we tell whether an action is a good action? Is it enough that we have good intentions? That the consequences of our actions are good? Or is there something more?

Moral Object, End of the Agent, and Circumstances

Catholic moral tradition holds that there are three sources of morality in human action: the moral object, the end of the agent, and the circumstances.[14] While these aspects can be found in each human action, they are not always easy to tease apart. Still, this approach offers us a useful tool for ethical analysis, and thus is helpful in discerning whether something is to be done or avoided.

The moral object is the action-in-itself, the deed to be done. John Paul II points out that of these three aspects, *"the morality of the human act depends primarily and fundamentally on the 'object' rationally chosen by the deliberate will."* [15] The moral object answers the question, what does the acting person choose to do? The moral object is that toward which the will aims. It is what is chosen.

While the moral object involves physical action, the two should not be confused. The moral object of an action, what we freely and consciously choose to do, is what can be either good or bad. Using a knife to cut open another person's chest is a physical action, but it can be good or bad depending on whether what is chosen is the performance of a needed surgery or the infliction of bodily harm. If the moral object is bad, then even the best intentions cannot make the act good. It is not licit to do evil that good may come of it (see Rom. 3:8). If the moral object is good or neutral, then we must next look to the intention of the moral agent and to the circumstances of the action in order to specify the morality of the act.

The end of the agent refers to the intention of the person performing the action. The end is something known only to him or her. The end answers the question, why does a person choose this moral object? Having good intentions is important, but if the moral object of an action is unworthy of our choice, then good intentions cannot make the action worthy. Take, for example, the case of a physician in dialogue with a terminally-ill twenty-seven-year-old father of two young children. The patient, who is mentally capable of making decisions and has always asked his physician to be honest with him, asks his physician to tell him whether he is likely to survive his disease. Even when asked frankly about the prognosis, the physician may be tempted to lie to the patient to protect him from the sadness of death. But to deceive a dying patient who is capable of making his own decisions and wants to know his prognosis is morally wrong, even if the physician might be upright in his aim. The physician's intention might be good (to protect the patient), but the moral object (lying to a patient who wants to know the truth) is problematic. The physician encumbers the patient's ability to make informed health care decisions, and in this case he also deprives the patient of an opportunity to prepare himself and his family adequately for his death.

If one were to choose a good moral object with a good intention (providing high-quality pain management to a dying patient out of a desire to relieve his physical burden so that he can spend time with his family), the good intention (relief of burden) would complement the good moral object (good palliation). A good intention cannot, however, make right an action that in itself is morally problematic. If one were to choose a good moral object with an evil intention (providing high-quality pain management in order to gain someone's trust, access his social security number, steal his identity, and drain his bank account), that evil intention would tarnish an otherwise good act. Both the moral object and the intention should be good in order for a human action to be good.

The *circumstances* answer the questions who, about what, by what means, when, where, why, and how. Responsibility and prudence demand that we consider the circumstances of our actions, including the likely consequences. *Consequences* refer to the goods obtained and the evils avoided as a result of a particular act. Consequences can make a good act better or a bad act worse, though they do not change the nature of the act itself. Giving alms to the poor is an act of charity, but if an intoxicated person asks for money while standing outside a liquor store, one might wonder if giving him money is the most charitable thing to do. If he says he wants cash to buy enough liquor to drink himself to unconsciousness, one might decide that giving money to this particular person at this time and in this place is not the most loving thing to do.

For a human action to be truly good, each of these aspects—the moral object, the end, and the circumstances—must be morally good. The human act is like an orchestra: all it takes is one out-of-tune oboe to create disharmony.

The traditional sources of morality in human action offer a helpful way to begin thinking through the aspects of morally relevant action. In the pages of this book, the authors will use analyses of these traditional sources of morality as applied to various topics, and will also introduce other bioethical principles that offer further guidance through case scenarios. Readers will soon see that some of the topics address questions to which the magisterium of the Church has offered clear, definitive teaching, whereas other topics venture into areas where Catholic Tradition offers principles and values to help shape a response but where a plurality of opinions or judgments may exist among those who are thoughtful and faithful.

The aim of this book is to provide insight into the way some bioethicists and moral theologians approach these topics from within the Catholic Tradition.

The Service of Bioethics

So why bother with bioethics?

For the parent in the pediatrician's office, bioethics offers criteria for making decisions about vaccination. For families discussing advance-care planning, bioethics offers a way of thinking through sometimes difficult end-of-life decisions, helping to reveal a range of morally legitimate options and ways to determine which option might be best in certain circumstances. In doing so, bioethics can provide peace of mind to those facing the end-stages of life and to loved ones making decisions on their behalf. For professionals in the workplace, bioethics offers a language that can be used to talk with colleagues about difficult choices in a way that is reasoned and respectful. Bioethics also helps health-care providers and scientists live out their professional vocations with integrity and in good conscience.

For some, bioethics is also a vocation, that is, a calling from God to a particular type of service—in this case, a professional service. The late Rev. Kevin O'Rourke, OP, one of the most influential Catholic bioethicists of our time, spoke of the vocation of bioethics as a service that helps others achieve some important goal. He likened the service of the bioethicist to Socrates's understanding of the service of the philosopher. Socrates spoke of the philosopher as the midwife, a midwife to the soul, since it is the role of the philosopher to help others discover truth. The philosopher does not step in and take over, Socrates thought, but helps a person discover truth on his own. O'Rourke held that a Catholic approach to bioethics, like that of Socrates's philosopher, is to serve as a midwife, to help people facing bioethical decisions make good and ultimately loving ones.[16]

Whether a person is a professional bioethicist, a member of a hospital ethics committee, a pastor, a counselor, a colleague, a family member, or a friend helping others make bioethical decisions, the work of bioethics can and should be a service of charity, an act of love, where the authentic good of others is the goal. The purpose of bioethics is to help us be the kind of people we were made to be: people called to love.

Notes

[1] Congregation for the Doctrine of the Faith (CDF), *Dignitas personae* (September 8, 2008), n. 10.

[2] *Catechism*, n. 1701; 2 Peter 1:4; John Paul II, *Evangelium vitae* (March 25, 1995), n. 2; and CDF, *Dignitas personae*, n. 8.

[3] See John Paul II, *Evangelium vitae*, n. 2.

[4] CDF, *Dignitas personae*, n. 8.

[5] C. S. Lewis, *The Weight of Glory* (New York: HarperOne, 2001), 46.

[6] John Paul II, *Fides et ratio* (September 14, 1998), n. 1.

[7] Antonio Spadaro, "A Big Heart Open to God: The Exclusive Interview with Pope Francis," *America* magazine, September 30, 2013, 24.

[8] See CDF, *Dignitas personae*, n. 37.

[9] See Vatican Council II, *Gaudium et spes*, Pastoral Constitution on the Church in the Modern World (December 7, 1965), n. 14.

[10] John Paul II, *Christofideles laici* (December 30, 1988), n. 38, emphasis removed.

[11] Vatican Council II, *Gaudium et spes*, n. 16, referencing Romans 2:15–16.

[12] Joseph de Finance, *An Ethical Inquiry*, trans. Michael O'Brien (Rome: Editrice Pontificia Università Gregoriana, 1991), 7.

[13] John Paul II, *Veritatis splendor* (August 6, 1993), n. 73.

[14] *Catechism*, n. 1750.

[15] John Paul II, *Veritatis splendor*, n. 78, original emphasis.

[16] Kevin O'Rourke, "Bioethics as a Vocation," presented at the Eighth Annual Conference on Contemporary Catholic Healthcare Ethics, Loyola University Chicago, October 9, 2009.

II

Assisted Reproductive Technologies

John M. Haas

Children ... are a gift from the Lord,
The fruit of the womb, a reward.
Like arrows in the hand of a warrior
Are the children born in one's youth.
Blessed are they whose quivers are full!
Ps. 127:3–5 NAB

These words from the psalmist speak eloquently of the goodness that children bring to life. The desire to bring offspring into the world is as old as Adam and Eve. Perhaps because of this, if childlessness seems to be one's lot in life, it brings its own particular heartache. A newly married couple looks forward not only to their life with each other but also to a life with those children who will be the fruit of their love. Indeed, they look forward to children as the incarnation of their love.

A newlywed husband and wife know that children bring challenges and sorrows as well as joys, but they look forward to these with a desire to complete the love they have sworn to one another. All young couples across time and cultures have known this eager anticipation. In ancient Israel, the priest Elkanah and his wife Hannah were much in love, but they were childless (1 Sam. 1:5). Even though they had one another, they longed for more; they wanted a child. But their desires were unfulfilled, and Hannah was disconsolate. Distraught himself, Elkanah said to his wife, "Hannah, why do you weep? And why do you not eat? ... Am I not more to you than ten sons?" (1 Sam. 1:8, RSV).

Of course she loved her husband, but Hannah wanted to see that love manifested in the children they had together. In this case, after time had passed, after many tears were shed, and after many petitions were offered to heaven, their prayer was heard and Hannah conceived. She gave birth to a boy who would become the prophet Samuel. But not all such prayers are answered as the couple would like. Some couples are called to embrace the cross of infertility.

It is perfectly understandable that couples desperately want to overcome their infertility. In a discussion of ethics, it is necessary to point out that not all means of assisting couples to have a child are morally acceptable. It is obvious that, morally speaking, the wife cannot sleep with another man, even though that has been done. There are also those who attempt to achieve pregnancy by having the wife artificially inseminated with the sperm from a donor.

Understanding the Child as a Gift, Not a Right

The Catholic Church teaches that parents do not have a "right" to a child. Such a right would make the child subordinate to the parents, as though he or she were their property. It would violate the personalist norm discussed in chapter 1: a person is an end in himself and not a means to an end. When a man and a woman marry, *they exchange rights to one another's bodies*; they give one another the exclusive rights to those actions which of their nature are appropriate to the engendering of children. The ordering of the conjugal life to the good of the spouses and the procreation and education of children is essential to marriage.[1]

The Church teaches that the child is a gift that arises out of the acts of love that the husband and wife show to one another. In other words, they are not to "use" one another even as they attempt to have a child. Marital relations between husband and wife are not a manufacturing process. A husband and a wife do not make babies. They make love with one another, and a child may or may not arise from those acts of love.

Regrettably, the incidence of infertility is at historic highs in the United States, and a veritable health care "industry" has arisen to help couples overcome their infertility. The Church understands and appreciates the desire of a married couple to seek assistance in overcoming their infertility but insists that some of the means being used today are simply beneath their dignity as human beings and do violence to their marriage and the martial act.

In 1987, the Holy See issued a document to assist married couples and their spiritual guides in evaluating the morality of certain means of overcoming infertility. Known as *Donum vitae*, or "The Gift of Life," it was produced by the Congregation for the Doctrine of the Faith under Cardinal Joseph Ratzinger. Its promulgation was approved by Pope St. John Paul II. It is often translated by its full name, which alludes to some of its basic themes: "Respect for Human Life in Its Origin and on the Dignity of Procreation." Its moral evaluations are as valid today as when the document was first issued.

Sorting through the various means of overcoming infertility can be daunting indeed. New means of overcoming infertility are continally being developed, and some are difficult to understand and evaluate morally. It should be made clear at the outset that the Church does not reject any means of overcoming infertility because it is artificial. Indeed, as stated in the introduction to *Donum vitae*, "These interventions are not to be rejected on the grounds that they are artificial. As such, they bear witness to the possibilities of the art of medicine."[2]

But the document does provide a "rule of thumb" that can be of assistance to couples trying to determine for themselves if a given technological intervention is or is not immoral. It is rather simple in its statement, but can be rather difficult to apply. If an intervention *replaces the marital act*, it is to be considered immoral, or beneath the dignity of the married couple. If it *assists the marital act* in achieving its natural purpose and end, that is, pregnancy, it might be moral.

In the words of *Donum vitae*, "If the technical means facilitates the conjugal act or helps it reach its natural objective, it can be morally acceptable. If, on the other hand, the procedure were to replace the conjugal act, it is morally illicit."[3] Let us see how this principle can be applied to certain means of overcoming infertility.

Fertility Drugs

Sometimes wives are unable to conceive because their eggs do not mature properly. Women of child-bearing age usually release one mature egg a month from alternating ovaries. Sometimes, however, assistance is needed with this process, and certain drugs can help. There is nothing inherently immoral about the use of drugs to stimulate ovulation. If more eggs are released, the chances are greater that one egg will be fertilized. One can see that the use of these drugs assists the marital act in achieving its natural end and does not replace it.

There are risks to such a procedure, however, and these should be carefully assessed. It could be wrong for a wife to place her health at too great a risk as she attempts to have a child. The use of hyper-ovulatory fertility drugs are sometimes not sufficiently regulated, and women may conceive four, five, or six children at once, causing considerable risk to their own health as well as to the health of the children they are carrying. Use of the drugs may also interrupt the normal development of the eggs, leading to unknown harmful consequences. Since the drugs cause eggs to mature more rapidly than they naturally would, they may interfere with genetic imprinting, which prepares the egg for fertilization and the engendering of a new and unique life.

Also, the use of fertility drugs is not without known dangers. Women have died from ovarian hyperstimulation syndrome. In 2002, the World Health Organization reported that 14 percent of women receiving fertility drug treatments suffered from this syndrome, with 1 percent being placed at risk of death.[4]

Furthermore, there is at times a terribly immoral procedure that takes place if the wife has conceived more children than she can safely carry to term. Doctors will propose an intervention known euphemistically as "fetal reduction." In this procedure, doctors monitor the development of the various fetuses and then destroy the ones that are least robust so that the mother only carries one or two of her babies to term. The others are killed by receiving an injection of potassium chloride into their chest cavity.

Along with the legitimate use of fertility drugs for women, one should also mention medications for men, such as Viagra. Sometimes the arteries in the penis do not allow sufficient blood flow for achieving an erection and performing the marital act. Certain drugs can overcome this problem. The effects of these drugs can last four hours (in the case of Viagra and Levitra) or up to 17.5 hours (in the case of Cialis). Because these drugs can have somewhat serious side effects, they can be obtained only with a doctor's prescription. The use of drugs that overcome erectile dysfunction could be morally licit for a husband, since they can help the marital act achieve its natural purpose.

Mechanical or Surgical Assistance

Sometimes surgery is required to remove blockages of the bodily tubes through which the sex cells pass, the vas deferens in the man and the fallopian tubes in the woman. At other times, the semen may have difficulty reaching the mouth of the uterus (the cervix) and can be assisted by a syringe or a cervical spoon. A vacuum constriction device may help the husband achieve and maintain an erection so that he can perform the marital act.

JOHN M. HAAS

It is not possible in this article to cover all the morally legitimate means that might be used to overcome infertility. But the few mentioned here indicate the proper application of the principle, or "rule of thumb," found in *Donum vitae*: if an intervention replaces the marital act, it is immoral; if it helps the marital act achieve its natural end, it may be moral.

Some techniques of overcoming infertility are not morally sound, because they do not promote the good of the couple or strengthen the couple's marriage. Careful analysis is critical, because many techniques touch in some way on innocent human life and on the God-given means by which children are to be engendered.

In Vitro Fertilization

One of the most common means of overcoming childlessness today is in vitro fertilization (IVF), literally "fertilization in glass." The children arising from this procedure are sometimes called "test-tube babies," but the fertilization actually takes place in a Petri or laboratory dish, not a test tube.

Many Catholics think the Church approves of this method, in the mistaken belief that the Church would support any method that helps a couple become pregnant. However, the Church rejects this procedure in the strongest terms, because IVF violates human dignity, marriage, and human life, as explained below. Despite its immorality, we must never forget that a child born by use of IVF is a child of God, to be loved and cherished as every child should be.

The process of IVF involves several steps. A number of eggs are aspirated from the wife's ovaries after she has taken a hyper-ovulatory drug. Semen is collected from the man, usually through masturbation. The gametes, or sex cells, are then joined in a Petri dish, where embryos develop for several days. An agreed-upon number of embryos are finally placed in the womb of the mother between one and six days after fertilization.

The process is immoral in several respects. The conception itself is extracorporeal—it takes place outside the wife's body—and this alone makes it immoral. In the words of *Donum vitae*, "Fertilization achieved *outside* the bodies of the couple remains *by this very fact* deprived of the meanings and the values which are expressed in the language of the body and in the union of human persons."[5]

It can also easily be seen that IVF *eliminates* the marriage act rather than helping it achieve its natural end. The new life is engendered by technicians in a laboratory rather than in the loving embrace of husband and wife. The husband and wife become merely the sources from which technicians collect the "raw materials" of egg and sperm and later manipulate them so that fertilization occurs. Not infrequently, eggs or sperm from a donor are used. This means that the father or mother of the child is someone other than the husband or wife. This can create a confusing situation for children later, when they realize that one of the parents raising them is not actually a biological parent. Perhaps the identity of the donor will never be known, depriving the child of an awareness of his or her own lineage—and also knowledge of health problems that could be inherited.

Even if the eggs and sperm come only from the spouses, there are still moral problems. Invariably, several embryos are engendered, and only those that show the greatest promise of growing to term are implanted in the womb. The others are discarded or are used for experiments. Some are frozen in liquid nitrogen for later use. In fact, it is estimated that more than six hundred thousand frozen embryos are being stored in the United States, most "left over" from IVF procedures.[6] The treatment of these embryos constitutes a terrible offense against human life. A beautiful little baby may indeed be engendered by IVF, but other lives are violated and often destroyed in the process.

The cost of the procedure can lead to other moral problems. In the United States one cycle of IVF costs, on average, $12,400 and has roughly a 20 percent success rate.[7] (Success rates are difficult to assess since they depend on so many different factors, such as the age of the wife or the condition of the lining of the womb.) Therefore, in a desire to hold down costs of the procedure and to increase the odds of success, doctors will sometimes transfer five or more embryos to the mother's womb to increase the likelihood of a successful pregnancy. But this sometimes results in more babies in the womb than the couple wants. To avoid this, doctors may perform a "fetal reduction," as previously mentioned, after monitoring the babies in the womb to see if they have any defects. If the babies are equally healthy, then the physician will simply eliminate the baby that is most accessible.

IVF therefore often involves unspeakable acts leading to the killing of nascent human life. But even if that does not occur, IVF still does violence to the marital act. As stated before, the marital act is not a manufacturing process, and children are not products. The marital act is one of mutual surrender in love. It is a total surrender of one's body, one's emotions, and one's powers of procreation. Through IVF, the couple eliminates the means by which God intends to engender new life, the act of love and surrender of a husband and a wife. In IVF, technicians are the ones who trigger the engendering of new life through their interventions, using the "raw materials" provided by the husband and wife.

Donum vitae recalls the true character of the marital act: "By its intimate structure, the conjugal act, while most closely uniting husband and wife, capacitates them for the generation of new lives, according to laws inscribed into the very being of man and woman."[8] Yet with IVF, children are engendered virtually through a "manufacturing process," they may be subjected to "quality control," and they may be eliminated if they are found to be "defective." We can see the dehumanizing dangers in some of these procedures by the very language used. Children are not engendered by technology or produced by an industry. Children are begotten, not made.

In the words of *Donum vitae*, "The connection between *in vitro* fertilization and the voluntary destruction of human embryos occurs too often. This is significant: through these procedures, with apparently contrary purposes, life and death are subjected to the decision of man, who thus sets himself up as the giver of life and death by decree."[9] The document speaks of "*the right of every person to be conceived and to be born within marriage and from marriage.*"[10] But "within and from marriage" means through the marriage act itself, which of its nature is ordered toward the transmission of life—and not by the manipulations of technicians.

Inherent in IVF is the danger of treating children, in their very coming-into-being as human beings, as somehow inferior to those who have engendered them, as products manufactured for the gratification of their parents. Even if one does not look on them in this way, the fact is that they are vulnerable and susceptible to the life-and-death decisions made about them by others as they come into being. As children are engendered through the marital act, they come into being in the hidden recesses of the mother's body, where they cannot be manipulated or rejected at the whim of others.

Another immoral intervention has developed from IVF. A technique known as pre-implantation genetic diagnosis (PGD) has been developed to allow medical personnel to extract a single cell from the human blastocyst in the Petri dish in order to test it and determine whether the blastocyst is defective or carries some genetic disorder. If judged to be defective, the blastocyst is destroyed. It is, literally, an act of eugenics on the microscopic level. The Germans, aware of their own sad recent history with eugenics, outlawed PGD in 2009, although that ban was partially overturned by a court decision in 2011.[11]

It is very important that couples avoid using IVF and that loved ones, friends, and relatives be dissuaded from making use of it. Often couples who have used IVF find themselves faced with terrible ethical choices that they never anticipated, such as deciding whether or not to use fetal reduction to eliminate some of the children they are carrying. They also often have to decide what to do with the frozen brothers and sisters of the children to whom they have already given birth. Should these frozen embryos be used for experimentation, destroyed, or given up for "adoption" to other infertile women? Couples using IVF frequently have no idea they will have to make such difficult decisions, none of which can be entirely moral.

Gamete Intrafallopian Transfer

Again, the most succinct statement of the principle that guides us in assessing the morality of interventions for infertile couples is that the intervention may not replace the marital act but may only assist it in attaining its natural end. One of the procedures that illustrates the difficulty of applying this principle is gamete intrafallopian transfer, or GIFT. In assessing this intervention, we will assume that those making use of it are married and that they engage in the marital act.

Before discussing the morality of GIFT, it should be pointed out that few if any fertility clinics will make use of it. It may be moral, but fertility clinics are interested in success rates they can advertise to draw more customers. GIFT simply does not have the success rate of IVF, so most physicians and clinics will not even offer it. If a couple pursues it and is able to find a clinic willing to offer it, however, it must still be morally evaluated.

In GIFT, ova are removed from the wife after she has taken a hyper-ovulatory drug. The couple engages in the marital act while the husband wears a condom with a perforation in the end. The condom is worn to procure the semen; the perforation allows some deposit of the semen in the vagina in order to complete the marital act.

Technicians remove the sperm from the semen and prepare them for the procedure. The sperm are placed in a thin catheter separated from an egg by an air bubble. The catheter is then placed in the fallopian tube, usually below a blockage, and the contents are deposited into the fallopian tube so that conception may occur in the body (in vivo) rather than outside it (in vitro).

Those who argue for the morality of GIFT claim that it merely assists the natural marital act that has already taken place. They maintain furthermore that it satisfies one of the conditions for the morality of infertility treatment specifically mentioned in *Donum vitae*, that is, that conception not take place outside the body.[12]

Those who argue against the morality of GIFT maintain that the actions that actually bring about the conception have *replaced* the marital act. The conjugal act is merely used as a means of collecting the male gametes. What brings about the conception is the intervention of the technicians using the gametes of the married couple. The simple fact that conception occurs within the body is not sufficient to render the procedure moral. Artificial insemination, even with sperm from the husband, replaces the marital act and is thus judged to be immoral despite the fact that conception occurs in the body.

The Holy See has made no definitive judgment on GIFT. Spiritual guides ought to provide couples with the arguments for and against its morality and leave them to make their own decisions.

Lower Tubal Ovum Transfer

Lower tubal ovum transfer is another fertility treatment that has not received a judgment from the Holy See, but no moral theologian considers it immoral. LTOT is usually performed when there is a blockage in the fallopian tube. As in GIFT, eggs are removed from the ovaries after the use of a hyperovulatory drug and are injected into the fallopian tube below the blockage. Normal conjugal intercourse takes place, and conception may or may not occur.

Surrogate Mothering

Another so-called reproductive technology that is sometimes used in the United States, but with less frequency than twenty years ago, is surrogate mothering.

Donum vitae describes the two kinds of surrogate mothering: (1) If the surrogate mother does not contribute her own ovum, she carries to term a child to whom she is a genetic stranger. (2) If she does contribute her own ovum, she carries the child of a man who is not her husband. In either case, she agrees to surrender the baby after birth "to the party who commissioned or made the agreement for the pregnancy."[13]

The procedure used in surrogate mothering is known as embryo transfer. The embryo is engendered in a Petri dish and then implanted in the uterus of the surrogate, who carries it to term. *Donum vitae* rejects the process as a violation against the child, for it deprives the child of its right to be conceived and born within the marital union of parents who have given themselves exclusively to one another.

In the United States, the term "surrogate mothering" usually refers to the second scenario, in which the husband of the infertile couple impregnates a woman other than his wife through artificial insemination. The so-called surrogate then carries the child to term and, after birth, gives the child up to the couple who contracted for her "services." She does this for a fee.

We can easily see how the marital union is violated in such an arrangement. We can also see that the so-called surrogate mother is the *actual* mother of the child, for she provides her own egg and is inseminated by another woman's husband. This arrangement is actually a species of adultery, since in marriage a husband and wife give each other exclusive rights to those actions which of their nature are apt for the generation of children. In surrogate mothering arrangements, those powers to generate life are not being used exclusively between the husband and wife. Furthermore, when the surrogate who donates her ovum is the actual mother, and she gives *her* child to the contracting couple for a fee, in a sense, she is selling her child to the contracting couple. When this arrangement was first used in the United States about thirty years ago, the Attorney

General of the state of Oklahoma voided all surrogate mothering contracts in the state because, he argued, they violated the state statute against trafficking in human flesh!

In surrogate mothering, the divine calling of parenthood is reduced to a commercial contract. The surrogate and the contracting couple draw up the terms of the arrangement at the beginning. The pregnancy is monitored. If the child is defective, the contracting couple can order the surrogate (remember, she is the actual mother) to abort the child. If she refuses, the contract is voided and she is left with full responsibility for the child—paying for the birth and postnatal care and raising the child herself. In such commercialization of childbearing there is also the danger of abusing poor women, since they could well be enticed into entering into such an arrangement in order to obtain money.

At the beginning of this chapter, a number of interventions were mentioned that are consistent with human dignity. At its conclusion, attention should be drawn to an organization that has committed its resources to helping couples overcome infertility ethically. Thomas Hilgers, MD, is the director of the Pope Paul VI Institute in Omaha, Nebraska. Pope Paul VI, of course, was the author of the 1968 encyclical *Humanae vitae*, which reiterated the Church's constant teaching on the immorality of contraception using contemporary language and concepts.

At the heart of the Pope's concern was the good of human life ("humanae vitae") within marriage, and the challenges raised to that good by contemporary attitudes and practices.

The Pope Paul VI Institute developed the Creighton Model FertilityCare System to help couples avoid or achieve pregnancies in ways that are fundamentally moral. Using the Creighton system, couples monitor the biological signs of fertility and make decisions based on a thorough understanding of the wife's cycle. Dr. Hilger's NaProTECHNOLOGY uses the same biomarkers to identify fertility problems and to correct them, providing medical and surgical intervention when required to correct the underlying conditions that cause infertility. Used by couples who have already tried IVF unsuccessfully, NaProTECHNOLOGY has reported substantially higher rates of successful pregnancy.[14]

Dealing with Infertility

Despite all the scientific advances and the prayers of infertile couples, some will remain childless. This will be a painful fact of life that the couple will have to endure. Friends and relatives should be sensitive and avoid being too inquisitive as to why they do not have children and should avoid suggesting that the condition may be due to some fault of their own.

Infertility is often particularly painful for the wife. John Paul II, in *Mulieris dignitatem*, points out that parenthood, in a sense, is realized more fully and intimately in the wife: "Although both of them together are parents of their child, the woman's motherhood constitutes a special 'part' in this shared parenthood, and the most demanding part. Parenthood—even though it belongs to both—is realized much more fully in the woman."[15]

But Christians are never simply to endure the crosses they encounter in life. We are called to embrace them, to make sense of them by offering them up to the Father in union with Our Lord's own offering on Calvary. We will never fully *understand* our crosses, but we can make sense of them by joining them to Christ's Cross for the benefit of others. As we read in the Catechism, "Spouses who still suffer from infertility after exhausting legitimate medical procedures should unite themselves with the Lord's Cross, the source of all spiritual fertility. They can give expression to their generosity by adopting abandoned children or performing demanding services for others."[16] They can also give themselves more fully to other family members or to their professional work for the benefit of others.

As Catholics, we are privileged to be part of a large and loving family. God has not left us orphans, or alone. When we are willing to embrace Christ as our greatest love and our highest good, then in return we "will receive a hundredfold, and inherit everlasting life" (Matt. 19:29).

Notes

[1] *Catechism*, n. 2201.

[2] Congregation for the Doctrine of the Faith (CDF), *Donum vitae*, Introduction, 3.

[3] Ibid., II.B.6.

[4] Jean-Noel Hugues, "Ovarian Stimulation for Assisted Reproductive Technologies," *Current Practices and Controversies in Assisted Reproduction*, ed. Effy Vayena, Patrick J. Rowe, and P. David Griffin (Geneva: World Health Organization, 2002), 114.

[5] CDF, *Donum vitae*, II.B.4b, emphasis added.

[6] In 2003, the number of frozen embryos stored in the United States was estimated to be nearly four hundred thousand. In 2012, the US government put that number at more than six hundred thousand. D. Hoffman et al., "Cryopreserved Embryos in the United States and Their Availability for Research," *Fertility and Sterility* 79.5 (May 2003): 1063–1069. Office of Population Affairs, "Embryo Adoption," US Department of Health and Human Services web site, 2012, http://www.hhs.gov/.

[7] American Society for Reproductive Medicine, "Frequently Asked Questions about Infertility," ASRM web site [undated], accessed January 28, 2013, http://www.asrm.org/.

[8] CDF, *Donum vitae*, II.B.4a.

[9] Ibid., II.A.

[10] Ibid., I.6, original emphasis.

[11] "German Parliament Allows Some Embryo Screening," *Spiegel Online*, July 7, 2011, http://www.spiegel.de/.

[12] CDF, *Donum vitae*, II.B.4b.

[13] Ibid., II.A.3.

[14] Thomas W. Hilgers, "Per-woman Pregnancy and Family Building Rates: NaProTECHNOLOGY and IVF," in *The NaProTECHNOLOGY Revolution: Unleashing the Power in a Woman's Cycle* (New York: Beaufort Books, 2010), 253.

[15] John Paul II, *Mulieris dignitatem*, n. 18.

[16] *Catechism*, n. 2379.

III

Vaccines and Abortion

Edward J. Furton

From choosing the perfect name to decorating the nursery, there is no shortage of thought that goes into decisions about the care of a precious new child. But there are also decisions that can be tough and may challenge the parents' sense of what is right and necessary for the health of their child. The subject of vaccinations falls into this category. Like many things, this subject does not touch us until a certain time of life, and then suddenly it looms large, and we must be informed. The decision to immunize a baby against childhood diseases is one that parents make early in the first year of their child's life. In this chapter we will look at one of the underlying moral issues concerning vaccines, specifically, how to deal with those that are associated with aborted fetuses.

Most people are unaware that a great many vaccines in common use today have an association with abortion. When they discover this hidden link, they are shocked and wonder how something like this could have happened. Even more importantly, they wonder about the proper course of action. They ask themselves if they should refuse to allow their child to be immunized with a vaccine made in this way.

Imagine that you are the mother of a young child who is about to enter first grade. Like all the other children, your child too must be given a shot against one or more contagious diseases, for example, the MMR vaccine which immunizes against measles, mumps, and rubella (German measles). Suppose that you now learn that this vaccine is grown in a cell line that originated in tissue obtained from an elective abortion. This discovery would be very distressing, because you would not want to have any association with the wrong of abortion. You would most likely be in a quandary about what you should do.

Suppose further that you decide, in good conscience, not to allow your child to receive the required immunization. You and your husband understand the benefits and the importance of immunization but have come to the conclusion that you cannot support the use of a product that has this type of origin. Having made your decision, you inform the school of your refusal. To your surprise, you then discover that the school will not admit your child to first grade.[1] The school policy is to admit only those children who have been properly immunized. Your child, therefore, cannot enter the first grade and must look for schooling elsewhere.

No child likes to receive a shot. Your decision against immunization might make your child very happy for the moment (he might be even happier to know that he cannot go to school), but you understand that there is a great deal more at stake here than a small amount of physical pain. The decision of the school not to admit your child to first grade presents a serious roadblock to education. If you look to other schools, you might find a similar policy in place. If all the schools in your area forbid the admission of a child who is not immunized, what can you do? Will you be charged with truancy or neglect if you do not enter your child into a recognized educational program? Will you be forced to homeschool your child?

Many states permit exemptions, either on religious or philosophical grounds (or both), but the difficulty for Catholics is that the Church does not offer religious grounds for objecting to the use of these vaccines. The Church's concern for the well-being of children takes precedence over the genuine moral concerns about cooperation with the past wrongdoing of others. The exemption on philosophical grounds offered in some states may enable Catholic parents to refuse on conscience grounds if they attend a public school, but an appeal to religious or philosophical objections is not likely to be successful in a Catholic school that is attentive to the Church's thinking in this area.

Source Text

The 2008 document *Dignitas personae*, issued by the Congregation for the Doctrine of the Faith, speaks of the problematic nature of these vaccines and offers us some direction:

> Grave reasons may be morally proportionate to justify the use of such "biological material." Thus, for example, danger to the health of children could permit parents to use a vaccine which was developed using cell lines of illicit origin, while keeping in mind that everyone has the duty to make known their disagreement and ask that their healthcare system make other types of vaccines available (n. 35).[2]

This judgment closely follows the reasoning in a 2005 article titled "Ethical Reflections on Vaccines Using Cells from Aborted Fetuses," whose author is the Very Rev. Angel Rodríguez Luño, a professor of fundamental moral theology at the Pontifical University of the Holy Cross in Rome.[3]

The topic at hand gives us an opportunity to explore and understand the principle of cooperation, a traditional tool of moral theology that is used to assess the culpability of those who in some way assist or benefit from the wrongdoing of another. The subject of categories of cooperation and their application was first developed by St. Alphonsus Liguori, founder of the Redemptorist order and a Doctor of the Church. He was particularly concerned about providing sound guidance to confessors, who were often confronted with difficult cases from penitents concerning whether they were committing sin by assisting another who was engaged in immoral conduct. Alphonsus lived at a time when there was a great struggle in the Church between the rigorists and the laxists, with the first group insisting on strict adherence to moral norms and the second arguing that it was more important to follow the spirit of the law than its letter. The approach taken by Alphonsus was to chart a middle path between these two extremes.

The Problem

In his article on vaccines, Rodríguez Luño takes note of the sad fact that some vaccines in current use have their origin in cell lines that were produced from aborted fetal tissue. In some cases, there are alternative vaccines that have no connection with abortion, but one must ask for them and they may not be immediately available. In some cases, there are no alternatives at all, so if one wants to have a child vaccinated, there is no other choice than using one of the compromised products.

How exactly did this problem begin? Rodríguez Luño only hints at the origins, but we can add some detail here. The first scientist to begin a human cell line was Leonard Hayflick, then a researcher at the

Wistar Institute in Philadelphia. Though the details are sketchy, Hayflick and his colleagues apparently screened women who planned to have an elective abortion, and afterwards removed some material (lung tissue) from the aborted fetuses and cultured these cells in the laboratory. The cells were made to proliferate, so that the original sample increased in size over time through duplication. Some of the cells were frozen for later use; others were allowed to continue to proliferate. These cells were then used in a variety of scientific research programs. In vaccine manufacture, these lines are used to grow attenuated live viruses which are injected under the skin to provoke an immune reaction. In some cases, the virus itself was also derived from an aborted fetus. Such was the case with the rubella virus strain RA 27/3, which was taken from an aborted child infected with rubella.[4]

There are several points of note here that will be important later when we examine the question of moral culpability. Here we must separate our heads from our hearts for a few moments, in order to ensure that the facts of the case are clearly in mind. Only then can we make a sound judgment about the moral question. In fact, the shock of discovering this connection may make it necessary to set aside further consideration of how to proceed until we have suffered through the emotions. Otherwise, any consideration of the facts will seem detached or lacking in the feelings that are proper to this discovery.

So let me emphasize, before proceeding to the facts, that the development of vaccines from aborted fetal tissue is a terrible injustice, not only for the children who were aborted and had cells removed, but also for parents who rightly want to have nothing to do with the practice of abortion—and yet find themselves confronted by this terrible dilemma.

First of all, we must bear in mind that these human cell lines duplicate themselves in the laboratory without the need for further abortions, so their use would not seem to increase pressure on women to have abortions. Second, the cells that are used in the manufacture of the vaccines are not those directly taken from the aborted child, but are "daughter" cells, that is, cells that have grown as descendants from the original aborted tissue. Third, after the vaccine has been grown in the problematic cell line, the manufacturer purifies the vaccine so that even these descendant cells are eliminated.

These factors already suggest that there are differing degrees of culpability on the part of the various individuals who come into contact with these cell lines. For example, the researcher who obtained the tissues from the aborted fetuses is obviously much more directly involved in the wrong of abortion than the physician who offers the purified vaccine to children in his office. Finally, following extensive research, there is no evidence that increasing exposure to the antibody-stimulating proteins and polysaccharides in vaccines in the first two years of life is related to the risk of developing autism spectrum disorder.[5]

Rodríguez Luño also notes that diseases such as rubella (German measles) pose a serious risk to public health. Rubella usually causes a rash on the face and neck that may spread to the rest of the body, but that typically lasts only two or three days. Teenagers and young adults may also experience swollen glands in the back of the neck and some swelling and stiffness in the lymph nodes. Most recover quickly from these symptoms without any aftereffects. The primary danger from rubella is to the unborn. A woman who contracts rubella while in the early stages of her pregnancy (the first eleven weeks) has a significant chance of miscarrying or giving birth to a deformed baby.[6]

The purpose of vaccinating young children against rubella, therefore, is not simply to protect them against the discomfort of a fairly mild childhood disease but, more importantly, to prevent infected children from passing the disease on to a pregnant woman and thus causing serious harm to her unborn child. The unborn may suffer serious birth defects or even death.

There are alternatives to the rubella vaccine that do not have any association with cell lines originating in abortion, but these products have not yet been approved for use in the United States. The irony is that if we wish to protect the future unborn by vaccinating against the ravages of rubella, we have no means of doing so except by taking advantage of the past unborn whose tissues were used to bring about the cell lines in which the inoculating vaccines were grown. Would the use of such a vaccine, when there is no alternative, be collaborating in the sin of another? Let us see.

Modalities and Degrees of Cooperation in Evil

We now move on to types of cooperating with evil: formal cooperation and material cooperation. These tools for moral analysis are useful with a great many moral questions that we confront in our personal lives and so are worth learning about even apart from the question of vaccines. The various distinctions, when you think about them, conform to what we would expect by common sense.

Formal cooperation occurs when someone shares the intention of the evildoer, that is, when he or she agrees with the wrongful action and provides assistance. It is easy to see that this type of cooperation is always wrong. Formal cooperators in the activity of counterfeiting, for example, would include those who help with the printing, stack the paper for use, add the ink to the machine, and agree to be paid in counterfeit bills. Those who contribute in this way are obviously a part of the gang and openly agree to participate in the wrong of counterfeiting itself.

Material cooperation occurs when someone does not share the same intention as the evildoer but none-theless contributes to the act for some other reason. This type of cooperation is not always wrong, and at times may even be justifiable, depending on the circumstances. For example, if counterfeiters kidnapped my wife and threatened to kill her unless I used my position at the United States Mint to obtain the needed paper, my reason for carrying out this action would not be to advance the cause of counterfeiting but to preserve the life of someone I love. Presumably, after she was released, I could then proceed to identify the culprits, and everyone would understand that this was a case not of formal cooperation but of justifiable material cooperation. Of course, if I did this same action to save my pet dog, I would not have a sufficient reason, and even my material cooperation would be wrong.

There are further distinctions among types of material cooperation. The first division is into immediate and mediate. As the names suggest, immediate cooperation is direct participation in the wrongful act itself (e.g., the act of counterfeiting) while mediate cooperation is not (e.g., supplying the paper for someone else to use in counterfeiting). Mediate cooperation is then divided into proximate and remote, the first signifying an action closer to the wrongdoing of another and the second an action further removed. Without getting too bogged down with the terms, what is important to see is that there are degrees of cooperation; some actions are more closely related to the wrongdoing, others less so.

The worse the evil that is being contemplated, the more one must seek distance from that wrong. Lesser evils may be tolerated, even if they involve closer association, if some other important good can be secured or evil avoided. Of course, one may never do wrong that good may come of it, so the act of the cooperator must be good in itself or at least indifferent (not necessarily either good or bad). Thus, a truck driver supplying surgical instruments to a hospital is in fact doing a good thing, even though he knows that some of those instruments will be used for abortions. The need to have a job and support his family, combined with the very limited nature of his involvement in the abortions, justifies this type of remote material cooperation.

Concerns about Tissues Obtained by Voluntary Abortion

In the United States, abortion has been declared a "right" by the US Supreme Court, which usurped the role of Congress by enacting legislation and imposing it on all fifty states. Many of our fellow citizens have grown accustomed to the destruction of human life. Many see nothing wrong with using aborted fetal remains that would otherwise, as they see it, "just go to waste."

Given these circumstances, we must mention yet another type of cooperation. In passive cooperation, one accepts the given situation as it is and refrains from making objections on the grounds that society has already changed so radically that any further protest is useless. The good Catholic, of course, will reject any active association with the taking of innocent human life, but that may no longer be enough. Today there is a need to oppose a wider culture that is willing to close its eyes to "structures of sin" that harm our common life together. Those who work in fields of research where fetal remains and human embryos are used as mere laboratory material have a special duty to speak out against these wrongs and to inform the public about them.

To understand the structure of sin more clearly, it is a good idea to pause here and visit the *Catechism of the Catholic Church*, which says this about the proliferation of sin:

> **1865** Sin creates a proclivity to sin; it engenders vice by repetition of the same acts. This results in perverse inclinations which cloud conscience and corrupt the concrete judgment of good and evil. Thus sin tends to reproduce itself and reinforce itself, but it cannot destroy the moral sense at its root.

> **1866** Vices can be classified according to the virtues they oppose, or also be linked to the capital sins which Christian experience has distinguished, following St. John Cassian and St. Gregory the Great.

They are called "capital" because they engender other sins, other vices. They are pride, avarice, envy, wrath, lust, gluttony, and sloth or acedia.

1867 The catechetical tradition also recalls that there are "*sins that cry to heaven*": the blood of Abel, the sin of the Sodomites, the cry of the people oppressed in Egypt, the cry of the foreigner, the widow, and the orphan, and injustice to the wage earner.

1868 Sin is a personal act. Moreover, we have a responsibility for the sins committed by others when we *cooperate in them*:

— by participating directly and voluntarily in them;

— by ordering, advising, praising, or approving them;

— by not disclosing or not hindering the when we have an obligation to do so;

— by protecting evildoers.

1869 Thus sin makes men accomplices of one another and causes concupiscence, violence, and injustice to reign among them. Sins give rise to social situations and institutions that are contrary to the divine goodness. "Structures of sin" are the expression and effect of personal sins. They lead their victims to do evil in their turn. In an analogous sense, they constitute a "social sin."

A researcher cannot plausibly argue that he is opposed to the destruction of human life and yet willingly accept fetal remains for his research work. Even though these lives were destroyed by others, he remains responsible in some measure for that wrong when he agrees to receive a benefit from the evil. His acceptance signals a willingness to participate in a wider culture that finds the taking of human life to be acceptable and seeks an advantage from what is a grievous wrong. So, too, do those in business who buy and market products created in this manner.

Ethical Considerations in the Use of Vaccines

Obviously, a person who uses a vaccine that has a distant origin in abortion is not the cause of that past evil act, but present use helps to foster the existing social malaise that sees human beings as fodder for programs of scientific research. To use the materials developed in this manner without expressing any moral concern is to give one's implicit approval (passive cooperation) to a system of research that is founded on what is evil. Hence, Rodríguez Luño contends that there is a clear moral obligation among physicians and parents to speak out against this mentality in society and to use whatever means are available to encourage social action that will counteract it.[7] We have a moral obligation to seek an end to the use of aborted fetal material and the destruction of human embryos in programs of scientific research.

There is a range of possible cooperation in connection with these vaccines and with the cell lines that are used to produce them. Those who freely accept intentionally destroyed human embryos or fetuses in their research are engaged in formal cooperation with an intrinsic evil; those in business who market these cells and the cell lines derived from them are engaged in mediate material cooperation; and those who use the vaccines, such as physicians and patients, engage in a remote form of mediate material cooperation.

Given these distinctions, we are now ready to answer our original question. What am I to do, as a parent, when I am confronted with the choice of whether or not to vaccinate my child? The answer is that I may allow immunization with these problematic vaccines and, indeed, if the disease is a serious one, I have a duty to do so. The reason is that the level of cooperation with the original wrongdoing is sufficiently remote, and the good achieved by vaccination is so great, that I ought to secure that good even though it remains connected to a very real but distant evil.

In *Dignitas personae*, the Congregation for the Doctrine of the Faith said, "Grave reasons may be morally proportionate to justify the use of such 'biological material.' Thus, for example, danger to the health of children could permit parents to use a vaccine which was developed using cell lines of illicit origin, while keeping in mind that everyone has the duty to make known their disagreement and to ask that their healthcare system make other types of vaccines available."[8] The article by Rodríguez Luño, which has been the focus of this series of reflections, is confirmed by this important Vatican statement.

The use of these problematic vaccines is material cooperation, but it is justifiable (1) because receiving a vaccination is itself a good act, and (2) because there is a sufficient reason for doing so in this problematic case, namely, because the failure to immunize poses a threat to the health of society, especially to those who are the most vulnerable among us. Thus, parents should immunize their children with these compromised vaccines when no alternatives are available, but they should do so "under protest" until such time as products without these immoral origins become available.

This conclusion would probably please Alphonsus, for we have arrived at a middle path between two extremes: we are not ready to use these products without any moral concern whatsoever, and we also would not refuse to use them and so put the health of others, children in particular, at risk. The devastating consequences of rubella, especially in the unborn, justify a minimal cooperation with the evil of abortion, but we must raise our objections to the wrongs that are being perpetrated by the research community. Obviously, placing parents in the position of having to choose between a compromised vaccine and an increased risk of disease is grossly unfair.

But the onus of this struggle cannot be placed on parents who have no other means of protecting their loved ones and society from the devastating consequences of these diseases. The parents have not asked that the vaccines be manufactured in cell lines that have an origin in abortion, and they have had no hand whatsoever in their production. They are simply presenting themselves at the appropriate time for their required immunizations. By expressing their objections to these products as they currently exist and by working to overturn this injustice against the unborn, they are doing what is morally required.

Thus, a parent who is confronted with the need to use a vaccine compromised by abortion should do so, and indeed has a moral obligation to do so, in view of the risks that follow from a failure to be properly immunized. The life and health of others, especially our children, take precedence over the minimal degree of cooperation that is at issue with an abortion which took place in the distant past and for which we bear no responsibility. At the same time, we must make strong efforts to counteract the growing tendency in pharmaceutical research and medicine to make use of tissues from intentionally destroyed human beings. We need to register our objections about a very clear structure of sin that is becoming a permanent fixture in the scientific community.

Given the above, it seems unlikely that a Catholic school would grant either a religious or a conscientious objection to immunization. Despite the strong moral reservations of some parents, these problematic vaccines guard against serious harms to students and their families. School administrators must follow the most appropriate course when considering how to effectively preserve the health of their students and their staff. Although there are no proper religious grounds for granting exemptions to immunizations, some Catholic schools may consider doing so on the grounds of conscientious objection. After all, one is bound to follow even an erring conscience. Yet school administrators also have a right of conscience, and they should expect that those who attend their schools have read and understood Church teaching in this area.

A Note on the Vaccine for Human Papillomavirus

And now we turn our attention to a subject that has caused some consternation to mothers of adolescent girls: whether to vaccinate against a particular sexually transmitted disease. The key difference between a vaccine offered against a contagious disease, such as rubella, and one offered against a sexually transmitted disease, such as human papillomavirus (HPV), is that the first is spread by involuntary means, such as coughing and sneezing, while the second is spread through voluntary sexual activity. Of course, some women are sexually assaulted. Others might be exposed to the virus when they marry men infected with it. There is nothing wrong with agreeing to be immunized against this disease so long as the product is effective.

But unlike other contagious illnesses, sexually transmitted diseases can be reduced through changes in personal behavior. Indeed, this would appear to be the best and first line of defense. The likelihood of contracting a sexual disease is directly proportional to the number of sexual contacts. The more contacts a person has, the higher the risk. It is that simple. Sexual abstinence and fidelity in marriage are the best protection against the harms that can be caused by promiscuous conduct.

Regrettably, some believe that serious moral problems, such as promiscuity, are best solved through technological means. They argue that researchers must provide us with a wide range of new vaccines that will immunize us against every conceivable type of sexually transmitted disease. In truth, however, moral problems need moral solutions, not technological ones. The most effective means of eradicating sexually transmitted disease is a willingness to respect the natural dignity and proper setting of human sexuality within marriage.

Governments, therefore, should not mandate immunization against sexually transmitted diseases, as this only addresses the effects of the problem and not its cause. Such mandates undermine the efforts of parents to instill sound moral conduct in their children.

Edward J. Furton

Frequently Asked Questions about Vaccines

Below are frequently asked questions about vaccines answered by ethicists from the National Catholic Bioethics Center.[9]

What is the Church's teaching about the use of certain vaccines that have a distant historical association with abortion?

There are a number of vaccines that are made in descendant cells of aborted fetuses. Abortion is a grave crime against innocent human life. We should always ask our physician whether the product he proposes for our use has a historical association with abortion. We should use an alternative vaccine if one is available.

What does it mean when we say that these products are made in "descendant cells"?

Descendant cells are the medium in which these vaccines are prepared. The cell lines under consideration were begun using cells taken from one or more fetuses aborted almost forty years ago. Since that time, the cell lines have grown independently. It is important to note that descendant cells are not the cells of the aborted child. They never, themselves, formed a part of the victim's body.

Vaccines and Abortion

How does one know when a particular vaccine has an association with abortion?

The cell lines WI-38 and MRC-5 are derived from tissue from aborted fetuses. Any product grown in the WI-38 and MRC-5 cell lines, therefore, has a distant association with abortion. The cells in these lines have gone through multiple divisions and replications before they are used in vaccine manufacture. After manufacture, the vaccines are removed from the cell lines and purified. One cannot accurately say that the vaccines contain any of the cells from the original abortion.

What does one do if a physician recommends one of these vaccines?

Sometimes alternative products, which are not associated with these cell lines, are available for immunization against certain diseases. For example, there is a rabies vaccine (RabAvert) and a single-dose mumps vaccine (Mumpsvax) that are equally safe and effective and do not have any association with abortion. You should ask your physician to use an alternative vaccine if doing so is practical, but there is no moral obligation to use a product that is less effective or difficult to obtain. Parents should check with their physician regarding the efficacy and availability of these and other vaccines.

Are there any vaccines for which there are no alternatives?

Unfortunately, at present there are no alternative vaccines available in the United States against rubella (German measles), varicella (chickenpox), and hepatitis A. All of these are grown in the cell lines WI-38 and/or MRC-5.[10]

What do I do if there is no alternative to a vaccine produced from these cell lines?

One is morally free to use the vaccine regardless of its historical association with abortion. The reason is that the risk to public health, if one chooses not to vaccinate, outweighs the legitimate concern about the origins of the vaccine. This is especially important for parents, who have a moral obligation to protect the life and health of their children and those around them.

What support is there in Church teaching for this position?

Dignitas personae, issued by the Vatican in 2008, holds that we may use these products, despite their distant association with abortion, so long as we protest their origins and ask for alternatives, at least until new, ethically developed vaccines become available.

Vaccines and Abortion

What can I do to ensure that alternative vaccines will be made available?

You can write to the pharmaceutical companies that make these products and insist that they manufacture vaccines that can be used by all without moral reservation. Also, you can contact your local legislators about your concerns.

Am I free to refuse to vaccinate myself or my children on the grounds of conscience?

One must follow a certain conscience even if it errs, but there is a responsibility to inform one's conscience properly. There would seem to be no proper grounds for refusing immunization against a dangerous contagious disease, for example, rubella, especially in light of the concern that we should all have for the health of our children, public health, and the common good.

Won't my use of these vaccines encourage others to destroy human life for research purposes?

Upon use, one should register a complaint with the manufacturer of the products as a form of conscientious objection. This signals opposition to the wider, morally reprehensible practice of using the unborn as little more than research material for science.

There is no moral obligation to register such a complaint in order to use these vaccines.

It should be obvious that vaccine use in these cases does not contribute directly to the practice of abortion since the reasons for having an abortion are not related to vaccine preparation.

Notes

[1] All but three states grant vaccine exemptions for school admittance based on religious beliefs; twenty states grant exemptions for philosophical, moral, or personal beliefs. National Conference of State Legislatures, "States with Religious and Philosophical Exemptions from School Immunization Requirements," July 6, 2015, http://www.ncsl.org/.

[2] Congregation for the Doctrine of the Faith, *Dignitas personae* (September 8, 2008), n. 35.

[3] Angel Rodríguez Luño, "Ethical Reflections on Vaccines Using Cells from Aborted Fetuses," *National Catholic Bioethics Quarterly* 6.3 (Autumn 2006): 453–459.

[4] College of Physicians of Philadelphia, "Human Cell Strains in Vaccine Development," *History of Vaccines* website, 2011, http://www.historyofvaccines.org/.

[5] Frank DeStefano, Christopher S. Price, and Eric S. Weintraub, "Increasing Exposure to Antibody-Stimulating Proteins and Polysaccharides in Vaccines Is Not Associated with Risk of Autism," *Journal of Pediatrics* 163.2 (August 2013): 561–567.

[6] The Centers for Disease Control and Prevention estimate that up to 90 percent of infants born to mothers infected with rubella in the first eleven weeks have a 90 percent chance of giving birth to a child with birth

defects, such as deafness, blindness, a damaged heart, an unusually small brain, or an intellectual disability. CDC, "Control and Prevention of Rubella: Evaluation and Management of Suspected Outbreaks, Rubella in Pregnant Women, and Surveillance for Congenital Rubella Syndrome," *MMWR Recommendations and Reports* 50.RR-12 (July 13, 2001): 1–23, http://www.cdc.gov/.

[7] Rodríguez Luño, "Ethical Reflections on Vaccines," 457–458.

[8] CDF, *Dignitas personae*, n. 35.

[9] Adapted from National Catholic Bioethics Center, "FAQ on the Use of Vaccines," 2006, http://www.ncbcenter.org/.

[10] Pontifical Academy for Life, "Moral Reflections on Vaccines Prepared from Cells Derived from Aborted Human Fetuses" (June 2005), reprinted in *National Catholic Bioethics Quarterly* 6.3 (Autumn 2006): 541–550, and available at http://www.ncbcenter.org/document.doc?id=7. See note 7 in that document for a list of alternative vaccines and their sources.

IV

Rape Protocols and Emergency Contraception

John M. Haas

The topic of emergency contraception in Catholic hospital protocols for rape victims might seem too complex and distant to be considered in a volume on Catholic moral teaching about bioethics. However, it is precisely because of the complexity of the issue, and because it has become a major topic in the area of public policy, that it is important for conscientious Catholics to understand what is at stake with respect to the free exercise of our religion and our deepest moral convictions.

The Catholic Church and Health Care in the United States

The Catholic Church has long been at the forefront of providing health care to those in need in the United

States. After government institutions, the largest
provider of health care in America is the Catholic
Church, with annual expenditures of more than
$100 billion. This vast ministry was begun mostly
by selfless, generous women religious who had left
everything to follow Jesus. They had given up any
possibility of having their own home, spouse, and
children for the sake of the Kingdom of God. They
placed themselves entirely at the service of God and
others. These women lived out the words of Pope St.
John Paul II in *Mulieris dignitatem*:

> Spiritual motherhood takes on many differ-
> ent forms. In the life of consecrated women, for
> example ... it can express itself as concern for
> people, especially the most needy: the sick, the
> handicapped, the abandoned, orphans, the elderly,
> children, young people, the imprisoned and, in
> general, people on the edges of society. In this way a
> consecrated woman finds her Spouse, different and
> the same in each and every person, according to His
> very words: "As you did it to one of the least of these
> my brethren, you did it to me" (Matt. 25:40). ...
> Spousal love—with its maternal potential hidden
> in the heart of women as a virginal bride—when
> joined to Christ, the Redeemer of each and every
> person, is also predisposed to being open to each
> and every person. This is confirmed in the religious
> communities of apostolic life.[1]

These religious sisters, many of whom were physicians, nurses, and founders of hospitals, showed
maternal love for all who came under their care, and
they served them with their spouse, Jesus Christ.

The health care ministry of the Church today is guided by the *Ethical and Religious Directives for Catholic Health Care Services* (*ERDs*) that have been issued by the United States Conference of Catholic Bishops.[2] These directives are in place to safeguard the dignity of all who are cared for in Catholic institutions. Medicine, like any human endeavor, has always required ethical guidance. Hippocrates, often referred to as the father of Western medicine, composed his ethical oath for physicians five hundred years before the birth of Christ. Unfortunately, in health care one may, driven by a sense of compassion, wish to do something for a patient that appears to help him in the short term but ultimately is not in his best interest.

The Victims of Sexual Assault

The former spokesperson for the United States bishops' conference, law professor Helen Alvaré, addressed the bishops on this terrible topic: "It is difficult for me to convey the horror of sexual assault. ... Rape reaches right to heart of a woman's feelings of physical vulnerability. It assaults her personhood, her womanhood, and conveys to her that she is just a thing to gratify someone else's violent impulses."[3] Professor Alvaré also pointed out that there is little awareness of what the Church does for victims of such violence.

In truth, Catholic health care has always shown particular solicitude to women who have been the victims of sexual assault. Indeed, Catholic hospitals were among the first to draw up specific protocols for the care these women should receive. Directive 36 of the *ERDs* calls for compassionate and understanding treatment of the victims of sexual assault and makes it clear that medical interventions to avoid pregnancy may indeed be ethically legitimate; they can be considered acts of self-defense:

> A female who has been raped should be able to defend herself against a potential conception from the sexual assault. If, after appropriate testing, there is no evidence that conception has occurred already, she may be treated with medications that would prevent ovulation, sperm capacitation, or fertilization. It is not permissible, however, to initiate or to recommend treatments that have as their purpose or direct effect the removal, destruction, or interference with the implantation of a fertilized ovum.

The Catholic Church wants to make certain that the woman is protected against the possible consequences of a sexual assault. The sperm of the assailant may legitimately be looked upon as an aggressor, and measures may be taken to try to prevent it from fertilizing an egg of the victim.

At the same time, the Church wants to make certain that it does nothing that would cause an abortion if a child has been conceived. The Church does not want there to be two victims of a sexual assault, the woman who has been violated and the child who may have been conceived before the assault or as a result of it. In treating the woman, the Church will not allow its institutions to do anything which may place in jeopardy a newly conceived life.

Directive 45 states clearly,

> Abortion (that is, the directly intended termination of pregnancy before viability or the directly intended destruction of a viable fetus) is never permitted. Every procedure whose sole immediate effect is the termination of pregnancy before viability is an abortion, which, in its moral context, includes the interval between conception and implantation of the embryo.

In the case of sexual assault, a contraceptive medical intervention as an act of self-defense is permitted, but abortion is not. This intervention to avoid conception is not the same type of contraceptive act that the Church has consistently taught is immoral. The act the Church has always judged to be beneath human dignity takes place when a married couple freely chooses to engage in the marital act but intervenes to thwart one of its purposes, procreation, from being realized.

The approach of the Catholic Church to victims of rape who are treated in its hospitals is one of compassion, understanding, balance, and reasonableness. The Church has been at the forefront in developing hospital protocols which provide direction as to how the victim may be treated to prevent pregnancy while avoiding abortion in the unlikely circumstance that conception has occurred. Catholic hospitals have always provided true emergency contraception to the victims of sexual assault.

Regrettably, there are enemies of Catholic health care because of the Church's position on contraception and abortion. There are those who are profoundly committed to making contraception and abortion universally available in health care institutions, and they view Catholic health care as contrary to women's best interests. The Catholic Church does not allow abortion or surgical sterilization in its hospitals because it considers them to be not true care for women's health but rather violations of a woman's physical, moral, and spiritual integrity. Abortion is particularly grievous, because it is the killing of a living human being. As mentioned above, directive 36 of the *ERDs* was put in place to help victims of rape defend themselves and avoid a possible abortion.

Rape Protocols

In practice, directives 36 and 45 can be difficult to apply. In 1995, Gerald McShane, MD, a physician with what is now OSF Saint Francis Medical Center, based in the Diocese of Peoria, Illinois, and the ethics committee of Saint Francis Medical Center developed a medical protocol that they believed would address the moral concerns contained in these directives, that is, self-defense for the victim and avoidance of an abortion. To understand the protocol, it will be helpful to outline briefly what happens before and during ovulation.

From basic human physiology, we know that a woman ovulates once a month from alternating ovaries. We also know that ovulation cannot occur unless certain hormones are present in the woman's body. These hormones can be measured. Each month there is a surge In luteinizing hormone (LH surge), which leads to the maturation and expulsion of the egg. An ovulation test can detect this hormone in the urine or, with greater accuracy, in the blood.

Dr. McShane reasoned that if it could be determined that the LH surge had not yet begun, the victim could be given a high dose of a hormone that would suppress the release of LH. This administered hormone would in effect be an anovulant, that is, it would prevent the woman from ovulating. If there were no egg present to be fertilized, the victim obviously could not and would not become pregnant. The use of these anovulant drugs can be viewed as so-called emergency contraception.[4]

The protocol for treating rape victims that Dr. McShane developed became known as the Peoria Protocol and was found to be morally permissible by the local bishop. From the beginning, some critics argued that the tests would not be accurate or that the actual mechanisms of anovulant drugs were not understood well enough to justify their use. In practice, the protocol has proved sound, allowing treatment decisions to be made with moral certainty.

The Virtue of Prudence

Medicine is as much an art as it is a science. Physicians often have to make their decisions on the medical evidence that they have available, on uncertain diagnoses, and on tentative prognoses. But they do the best they can. Prudence is the moral virtue that enables everyone, physicians included, to make the best decisions possible in concrete situations with the information available. Prudence is considered the highest of the moral virtues because it gives us the capacity to look at reality for what it is and weigh the facts objectively. St. Thomas Aquinas called prudence the "mother of all virtues."[5] With prudence, we make a decision to act here and now, which, ultimately, is what the moral life is all about.

Some people want absolute certitude that their decision is the right one. But because of the human condition and our inability to know everything, we cannot always have absolute certitude—and that should not keep us from acting. In fact, prudential certitude is precisely the kind of certitude that one uses in making moral decisions, even life-and-death ones, although in such cases the greatest effort must be made to eliminate as much doubt and ambiguity from the situation as can be reasonably expected. Prudential certitude is the type of certainty that is used in ethical decision making; it takes full account of the ambiguities of human knowledge arising from our finitude and from the virtually endless circumstances that surround any human act.

With respect to the Peoria Protocol, there would certainly seem to be enough evidence from urine or blood tests indicating the occurrence (or absence) of the LH surge to enable one to make a decision about whether one ought to use a particular drug to suppress ovulation and avoid pregnancy.

The Risk of Abortion and Rape Protocols

Health care professionals looking after the victim of a sexual assault want to help her protect herself from the sperm of her assailant, but they do not want to initiate any intervention that would lead to the "removal, destruction, or interference with the implantation" of a child who has already been conceived (directive 36). The morality of the use of emergency contraception has already been discussed. However, the mechanisms of the drugs used as emergency contraception may well have other properties that make their use morally problematic, particularly with respect to the timing of their use.

How do these drugs work? Most experts point to other effects of these commonly used drugs which go beyond preventing ovulation. The drugs may affect the consistency of the mucus at the opening of the womb, which makes it more difficult for the sperm to get through. But what can raise true ethical problems is the possibility that the drugs prevent a new life from implanting in the womb. The question is, if a drug is administered too late to prevent ovulation and if the woman conceives, does the drug prevent the implantation of that new life in its mother's womb? If it does, the drug has an abortifacient rather than contraceptive effect. To use a drug as an abortifacient would indeed violate directives 36 and 45, because it places in jeopardy a new human being who might have already been conceived.

It is for this reason that some moralists and physicians object to any use of emergency contraceptive drugs whatsoever, whether prior to ovulation or after it: if the findings of an ovulation test are not correct, if a mistake has been made about ovulation not having occurred and a child has been conceived, the drugs may have an abortifacient effect. There is also considerable dispute over whether or not emergency contraceptive drugs *ever* have abortifacient effects. The scientific debate is far too complex for this article. However, if the focus of the administration of the drug is on preventing ovulation, the debate over whether or not it may also have an abortifacient effect would not be an issue.

Another difficulty with the protocol is that there is no way to determine right away whether or not a woman has conceived from the rape. Directive 36 speaks of the need to administer certain tests before intervening with medications: "If, after appropriate testing, there is no evidence that conception has occurred already, she may be treated with medications that would prevent ovulation, sperm capacitation, or fertilization."

"Appropriate testing" cannot refer here simply to a test to determine whether conception occurred following the rape, since no test will tell us that. An ovulation test will show whether a pregnancy occurred prior to the rape *or* whether the woman has ovulated (and hence whether or not anovulant drugs might "prevent ovulation, sperm capacitation, or fertilization"). But no test can tell us right away whether a new human being has come into existence as a result of the rape. Anovulant drugs should be given within seventy-two hours of the rape, before it can be known whether a woman has conceived.

A new life is conceived in the fallopian tube, or oviduct, which then travels for five days down to the womb of the mother. There it will implant in the wall of the uterus, putting down "roots," known as chorionic villi, to draw nourishment from the mother. The chorionic villi secrete a hormone known as human chorionic gonadotropin, or hCG. This hormone is what is detected in the urine or blood and indicates that a woman is pregnant. However, this hormone usually appears in the blood or urine of a pregnant woman about ten days *after* she has already become pregnant. Therefore, when a pregnancy test is administered to the victim of rape and the result is positive, the test tells us nothing about the consequences of the rape but only that the woman was pregnant prior to the rape. Obviously, the administration of a drug to suppress ovulation would be mindless in such a case, since the woman is already pregnant. The only effect the drug would have is a possible adverse one on the developing child.

Immoral Government Mandates

Into this very complex and sensitive issue step the abortion lobby and several state governments. There are pro-abortion groups in the United States that have seized on directive 36 as a way of pushing their own agendas. They have pointed out that the Catholic Church itself allows emergency contraception in cases of rape. However, they then turn to the government to force Catholic institutions to administer these drugs without administering the appropriate tests to see whether the drugs will have their intended effect.

Clearly, Catholic hospitals will not want to administer a drug to stop ovulation if ovulation has already occurred. These drugs must be given in high doses, and they have some unpleasant side effects. Why would a physician give an anovulant, a drug to suppress ovulation, without administering a simple test to see if the drug will even have its desired effect?

One reason must be that these organizations know that the drugs may also have the effect of preventing a new life from implanting in the womb, which the organizations are willing to see happen. Their intent is to force Catholic health care institutions to engage in interventions that might prove to be abortifacient, with no regard for the consciences of Catholic health care institutions and with no regard for what these institutions consider to be good medicine in the interests of their patients.

Mandates in several states require Catholic institutions to give these medications to rape victims upon request whether or not the victim is ovulating and whether or not a child has already been conceived. Some states (e.g., Massachusetts) are so overbearing in their demands that they do not allow a hospital even to require a pregnancy test to determine whether the woman was pregnant prior to the rape.[6] Other states may allow a pregnancy test but make it illegal to require an ovulation test.[7] These prohibitions are simply bad medicine, and they make use of the devastating circumstances of victimized women to advance the agenda of the pro-abortion lobby.

Even though the ultimate agenda of these organizations is to advance access to abortion, they confuse the issue by referring to their demands as the provision of emergency contraception. When a state Catholic conference opposes passage of such a law, it is portrayed as being insensitive to rape victims and opposed to emergency contraception. In cases of rape, however, the Church has always supported and provided emergency contraception, but not "emergency *abortion*," which, again, is the objective of these groups.

A typical example of the politicization of health care is the Massachusetts law that mandates emergency contraception.[8] In truth, the mandate is not directed at emergency contraception but at emergency *abortion*, since the mandate forbids testing to see whether the medication will work as a contraceptive or an abortifacient.

A circular letter issued by the Massachusetts Department of Health and Human Services dated June 27, 2008, holds that a hospital cannot state that "emergency contraception" is "contraindicated if an ovulation test is positive."[9] In other words, an emergency room cannot administer a test to see if a woman has ovulated and tell her that, if she has already ovulated, it would be medically inappropriate to administer a drug that would not achieve the purpose for which it was being administered. In other words, hospital personnel may not give the victim of rape all the information that pertains to her treatment and must, instead, provide her with information written by the Massachusetts Commissioner of Health. It is surely a violation of the dignity of women to withhold information about all the ramifications of a proposed medical intervention. It denies women their right to know all the facts simply because those who urged the passage of the law do not consider interference with the implantation of a new life in the womb of the mother to be immoral.

Regulations such as these from the Massachusetts Department of Health and Human Services also make it abundantly clear that the target of this legislation is Catholic health care; other institutions do not administer an ovulation test. Again, they do not administer an ovulation test presumably because they have no moral qualms about the possibility of causing a chemical abortion.

The regulations go so far as to make certain that the religious beliefs and moral convictions of health care professionals cannot interfere with the administration of any emergency contraception medication that the victim requests. The regulations state specifically, "To ensure that particular hospital staff's values or beliefs do not interfere with compliance with the law, the hospital will institute systems to ensure that all female rape victims ... are promptly offered emergency contraception, and emergency contraception is initiated upon her request." [10]

Many women are health care professionals or hospital administrators. Through laws and regulations such as these, they are denied the ability to make their own decisions based on their best medical judgments with regard to the treatment of patients. Once again, if a woman has ovulated, why, medically, would she be offered a medication to prevent ovulation? Why, legally, would the state prohibit even the administration of a test to see whether or not she has ovulated? Since when do the patients determine and insist on being given a particular drug without the advice or consent of a trained health care professional? We can see here how an ideology that is supposedly committed to advancing women's rights can actually work against women. When an idea turns into an ideology, it no longer considers the facts. Rather, it is driven by another goal to which human beings are subordinated.

Plan B One-Step

Plan B One-Step is the brand name of a hormonal agent that is used as a "backup" measure to "prevent pregnancy after birth control failure or unprotected sex."[11] ("If Plan A fails, use Plan B.") It is manufactured by Teva Women's Health, a subsidiary of Teva Pharmaceuticals, and consists of one dose of the hormone levonorgestrel, which is a synthetic form of progestin, the same ingredient often used in regular birth control pills. The original Plan B consisted of two 0.75 mg doses of levonorgestrel taken twelve hours apart, but Plan B One-Step is a one-pill, 1.5 mg dose of the hormone. The manufacturer directs that, to be effective, it should be taken within seventy-two hours of sexual intercourse.

Every other kind of oral contraceptive requires a prescription from a competent, licensed health care professional. This is because hormonal agents can interfere with the normal functioning of the body and may interact badly with other medications. However, there was a major political battle to get Plan B approved by the Food and Drug Administration for distribution without a prescription. This was finally achieved for women eighteen years old and over in 2006. In 2013, Plan B One-Step was made available to minors without a prescription as well. This sets Plan B One-Step apart from any other kind of birth control medication and again demonstrates the desire to make medications that may be abortifacient available as widely as possible. As with other medical matters, what is supposed to be in the best interest of women may in fact work against their best interest. For example, a man guilty of statutory rape may compel the young woman to take emergency contraception to counter the consequences of his actions.

The fact that Plan B is available without a prescription has also been incorporated into the mandated rape protocols in Massachusetts. The regulations state, "When providing Emergency Contraception, the hospital offers pills (i.e., not a prescription)."[12] The fact that Plan B and Plan B One-Step are available without a prescription does not help the Catholic health care institution avoid being complicit in their administration. Even as over-the-counter drugs, they cannot be given in the emergency room of a hospital without the consent of the emergency room physician or nurse supervisor. This means the Catholic hospital must cooperate in the distribution of a drug it may consider useless (in not preventing ovulation) or destructive (in preventing the implantation of the embryo).

How Plan B and Plan B One-Step work is still being studied, and findings are inconclusive. The manufacturer, the Food and Drug Administration, the *Physicians' Desk Reference*, and the American College of Obstetrics and Gynecology all state that levonorgestrel appears to work by (1) preventing ovulation, (2) inhibiting fertilization because of its effect on the cervical mucus, and (3) preventing the implantation of an embryo. It is the third probable effect that causes Catholic health care professionals such concern. And Catholic hospitals have tried to reduce the risk of that happening by providing the ovulation test to the victims of sexual assault.

The Need for a Well-Formed Conscience

It is obvious that the ethical use of emergency contraceptives in Catholic hospitals is a very complex question. There are different ways in which bishops across the country have addressed the problem. Some bishops insist that their hospitals administer an ovulation test before giving emergency contraception, and some do not. Also, mandates on providing emergency contraception vary in significant ways from state to state. However, it is important for Catholic laity to be well informed about challenges to Catholic morality and to develop well-formed consciences about contemporary issues. In matters as complex as these, it is important to keep in mind that the basic, fundamental concern of the Church in her health care ministry is always the dignity and worth of every human being, created in the image and likeness of God and redeemed by Jesus Christ.

Notes

[1] John Paul II, *Mulieris dignitatem*, On the Dignity and Vocation of Women (August 15, 1988), n. 21.

[2] United States Conference of Catholic Bishops, *Ethical and Religious Directives for Catholic Health Care Services*, 5th ed. (Washington, DC: USCCB, 2009).

[3] Helen M. Alvaré, "The Prevention of Pregnancy after Sexual Assault," in *Urged On by Christ: Catholic Health Care in Tension with Contemporary Culture*, ed. Edward J. Furton (Philadelphia: National Catholic Bioethics Center, 2007), 144.

[4] For a thorough and scientific discussion of this protocol, see Edward J. Furton, ed., *Catholic Health Care Ethics: A Manual for Ethics Committees*, 2nd ed. (Philadelphia: National Catholic Bioethics Center), 2008.

[5] Thomas Aquinas, *Scriptum super libros sententiarum* III.33.2.5 (Bologna: Edizioni Studio Domenicano, 2000), 6.652.

[6] "Every patient or resident of a facility shall have the right ... if the patient is a female rape victim of child-bearing age, to receive medically and factually accurate written information prepared by the commissioner of public health about emergency contraception; to be promptly offered emergency contraception; and to be

provided with emergency contraception upon request." Mass. Gen. Laws ch. 111, § 70e.

[7] In Connecticut, for example, the law states that "no licensed health care facility that provides emergency treatment to a victim of sexual assault shall determine such facility's protocol for complying with the standard of care requirements prescribed [here] on any basis other than a pregnancy test approved by the United States Food and Drug Administration." Conn. Pub. Act 07–24, SB 1343.1(b)3(d) (May 16, 2007).

[8] Mass. Gen. Laws ch. 111, § 70e (o); Session Laws 2005 ch. 91; and regulations 105 CMR 130.1040–130.1043.

[9] Mass. Health and Human Services, circular letter DHCQ 08–06–492 (June 27, 2008), attachment B.

[10] Ibid., attachment A.

[11] Plan B One-Step FAQ, July 2013, http://www.planb onestep.com/, accessed September 16, 2013.

[12] Mass. HHS circular letter, attachment A.

V

ORGAN TRANSPLANTATION

Edward J. Furton

Organ donation has become a common practice, and many people know or have met someone who either has donated an organ or has received one. Pope St. John Paul II, in his encyclical *Evangelium vitae* (The Gospel of Life), described organ donation as a form of moral heroism that builds the culture of life: "A particularly praiseworthy example of such gestures is the donation of organs, performed in an ethically acceptable manner, with a view to offering a chance of health and even of life itself to the sick who sometimes have no other hope" (n. 86).

The United States Conference of Catholic Bishops provides guidelines for organ donation by living donors as well as for donation after a donor's death. Living donation may be as simple as giving blood under the supervision of a nurse or as complex as whole organ transplantation under the medical expertise of a team of specialists. In living organ donation, the central moral concerns are that the donor makes an informed decision, does not suffer any loss of functional integrity, and gives the donation as a true gift, not as an exchange for money. The main moral concern in donation after death pertains to the physician's determination that death has in fact occurred.

Living organ donation initially posed a puzzle for theologians. Church teaching forbids the mutilation of the body except when it is necessary for the greater good of the entire person. For example, one may remove a gangrenous leg if doing so will save the life of a patient; the good of the parts are ordered to the good of the whole. But when we donate an organ to another person, it would seem that we mutilate our own bodies without any clear advantage to ourselves. The act of donation greatly benefits the other person and may even save a life, but how can one justify the mutilating loss of an organic part, even for a good cause? What right do we have to intentionally damage our own bodies?

After an initial period of uncertainty, theologians generally responded in favor of organ donation with two essential points. First, the gift of an organ is an act of charity, they said, and therefore is praiseworthy when properly performed. We are free to make sacrifices for others in the spirit of Christ, even if those sacrifices may cause some harm to ourselves. Yet this reasoning, sound as it is, does not justify any type of self-inflicted harm. Perhaps someone I love has a failing heart. My willingness to sacrifice for another would not justify the removal of my own heart, as that would bring about my immediate death. Suicide is a type of unjust killing.

A second argument in favor of organ donation allows that not all types of physical mutilation constitute functional mutilations. The loss of a single kidney, for example, does not harm the functional integrity of the whole body, which can continue to purify the blood with the remaining organ. Yes, there is indeed a mutilation, but it does not affect the integrity of the body as a functional whole. Because the kidneys are paired, the act of donation is justified in an act of charity. But this is not true with all paired organs. The eyes are also paired, but because the loss of an eye would result in a very obvious diminishment in vision, that type of donation remains immoral. Indeed, even the donation of a cornea (the outer layer of the eye) would adversely affect one's vision as a whole. Functional integrity would not be maintained.

Some single organs may also be donated in part. The liver, for example, will grow back after the live donation of a portion.

Outside the Catholic Church, some have argued that the bodies of anencephalic children (who have only a functioning brain stem) may be used for the retrieval of organs. They take this view because they do not consider these children to be human beings. Some parents may be tempted to think that the child does not have a life worth living and therefore organ donation might at least achieve some good. Yet these children are indeed human, even though they have suffered a terrible birth defect. Should the child expire, then organs may be taken following an appropriate determination of death by a physician. We may never kill another human being for organs, even though it might be of benefit to another.

The 2000 Address of John Paul II

John Paul II's Address to the Eighteenth International Congress of the Transplantation Society, delivered in August 2000, sums up a number of key moral questions concerning organ donation.[1] This short speech remains among the best summaries of Church teaching on the dangers of commodifying the body, the need for informed consent, the challenge of properly determining death, the use of neurological (brain death) criteria, the just allocation of scarce organs, and xenotransplantation (the transplantation of organs from animals to human beings).

Of these topics, brain death undoubtedly remains the most controversial. Surprisingly, the foundation for the Church's response was first laid out by Pope Pius XII in his Address to an International Congress of Anesthesiologists on November 24, 1957.[2] There he enumerates several key principles that would guide later teachings, affirming, for example, that it is the responsibility of the physician to determine the moment of death. The Catholic Church defines death as the separation of the spiritual soul from the material body, but it relies on the judgment of physicians to determine when that event has occurred. But let us look at each of these important issues in their proper order.

No Commercialization of the Body

First, John Paul II reminds us of the central point that "the integral good of the human person" is the guiding truth in all deliberations concerning the appropriateness of any medical procedures.[3] The word "integral" reminds us of the principle of totality and integrity touched on above, which demands that we see the human body as an organic whole whose parts are ordered to the good of the entire person. An organ forms a part of the body and thus a part of the body-soul union that is the person. We express our personhood through our bodies; hence, the decision to give a part of one's own body to another constitutes a unique gift of self and a profound act of love.

The gift of organ donation must be made without monetary advantage. How else would it be a gift or a donation? Of course, one should be reimbursed for one's time and expense. Typically, the cost of the hospital stay and the surgical operation is covered by others, but it is reasonable to expect compensation for loss of time at work and other incidental expenses. But beyond that, it would not be right to accept financial reward. To receive money in exchange for an organ is to turn the body into an article of trade and thus to treat it as if it were a mere object of use. This makes the body into a thing, but the body is the subjective sphere of our personhood, completely unique to each individual and incapable of becoming a commercial product. To sell an organ is dehumanizing.

The sale of organs has become a serious problem in our modern global culture. The citizens of poorer countries often accept the prospect of easy money and allow a surgeon to remove a healthy organ for a buyer. Although John Paul II does not directly address this problem, as no respectable transplant surgeon in his audience would have stooped to such a practice, the Church's rejection of buying body parts from the poor follows from his observation that the sale of human organs violates the intrinsic dignity of the human person. Trafficking in organs nonetheless continues to grow, with some attempting to justify the practice as mutually beneficial for all concerned. Catholics must fight against the growing commercialization of the body.

Ascertaining the Fact of Death

It is "self-evident," John Paul II says, that we can never bring about the death of another human being in order to acquire an organ for transplantation. Certainly, no sensible person can deny this. Thus, we can never remove "vital organs which occur singly in the body" until after the death of the donor.[4] In order to ensure that the removal does not cause or contribute to the death of the donor, we need to be certain that death has already occurred before the organ is taken. Though it is often obvious that a person has, in fact, died, there are cases in which this is not immediately apparent. Society has assigned the task of determining death to the physician, who has the medical expertise to carry out this critically important function. The Church is ready to follow the legitimate standards of determining death that have been established within the medical profession.

Nonetheless, there are certain truths about death that are unavailable to medicine, but that have been discovered instead through the Church's philosophical tradition. Death is the separation of the soul from our earthly existence, where "soul" means the principle of life that animates the body. This insight into the nature of death is drawn from the most ancient sources in the Church's intellectual tradition and is also connected to important observations about the nonmaterial (spiritual) character of the soul. Also, death occurs at a moment in time, namely, at the moment of separation. The soul does not cease to exist at death, but continues to dwell in the afterlife, sustained by God, as it awaits the resurrection of the body.

John Paul II engages these deeper metaphysical truths about death and the human person when he reaffirms the earlier statement by Pius XII that the moment of death is not directly observable.[5] Death is not an empirical event. Instead, we experience our own death as a departure from the body, and this interior experience will always be hidden from science. What the physician sees instead are the external signs that death has occurred. On the basis of these external signs, the doctor rightly pronounces death. Thus, the determination of death depends on knowing the appropriate external signs.

The Use of Neurological Criteria

There are essentially two methods of determining death: the traditional cardiopulmonary method and the newer neurological, or brain death, method. The first looks to the cessation of heartbeat and the loss of circulatory function. This has been the primary means of determining death throughout history. In contrast, brain death looks to the electrochemical activity within the skull. Both have generated controversy, but the second is the more hotly contested because those who suffer brain death may still have cardiopulmonary function.

The cardiopulmonary method would seem to be very clear, but the eagerness of transplant specialists to harvest organs leads to questions about how much time must pass before one can declare that the patient has indeed died. This must be assessed with great care if we are to avoid any possibility of contributing to the death of the donor. Typically, the physician waits five minutes after asystole (cessation of heartbeat) on the assumption that spontaneous resuscitation of the heart is impossible after that time. This seems a reasonable standard; however, others have sought to shorten this time, some to as little as two minutes. This shortening is troubling, but has found wider acceptance in recent years. Five minutes seems a more reasonable standard, as it is obviously best to err on the side of caution. The transplant community should realize that if it breaks trust with the public and frightens organ donors, its effort to acquire more organs by cutting corners will backfire.

The neurological criteria for the determination of death are, in some ways, a more certain standard than the cardiopulmonary ones, but they, too, pose challenges. Here, one must recognize that the brain plays the dominant role in organizing the physical body, and that the soul exercises its primary functions in a unique way via this central, unifying organ. All sensory and cognitive functions originate and terminate in the brain. The brain stem is the vital passageway for the autonomic functions of the body.

These medical facts correspond well to the Catholic teaching that the human being is a unity of body and intellective soul, that is, a soul blessed with the capacity for intellectual thought. This ability is not given to any other creature and is the special mark of our human nature.

When the entire brain, including the brain stem, lacks function, the person is dead. Such is the general judgment of the medical community. Given this medical judgment, and given Catholic teaching on the nature of the soul and death, the "whole brain" standard of determining death corresponds to what John Paul II calls "the Christian understanding of the unity of the person."[6] We are created by God to be rational creatures; when our intellectual function has permanently ceased, we may properly conclude that death has occurred. John Paul II therefore concludes that neurological criteria may be used by health care workers and their patients when making decisions about the donation of organs.

John Paul II does not give unqualified approval to this method of determining death, but says instead that it "does not seem to conflict with the essential elements of a sound anthropology."[7] The work of the Church is to provide guidance concerning good and right human actions, not to offer technical advice about medical standards. Given the "clearly determined parameters commonly held by the international scientific community," and presuming these criteria are "rigorously applied," John Paul II affirms that neurological criteria provide us with sufficient "moral certainty" to be confident that we act rightly if we give, receive, or assist with organ transplantation under this medical standard.[8]

Moral certitude was discussed in chapter 4. As noted, we cannot have the same degree of certitude in morals as we can expect to have in other sciences. For example, I can know with complete certitude that 2 + 2 = 4, but I cannot know with the same level of certitude whether I should see a doctor about a cough, correct a colleague about an inappropriate comment, or speak to a neighbor about a political campaign. Life confronts us with many moral questions, and we cannot expect to have complete assurance that every choice will always be the best, nor does the Church require this. We can only try to form our consciences as best we can in the light of the available facts, and make our best decision. If we waited for perfect moral certitude, we would often be unable to act at all. The neurological criteria, John Paul II says, provide us with sufficient certitude for action.

Controversies over Neurological Criteria

Neurological criteria are controversial because the body continues to show signs of life after the declaration of death. Most remarkably, both respiration and heartbeat continue, though this only happens through the application of mechanical means of support. Once the external apparatus is removed, these movements cease. Opponents of brain-death criteria are very uneasy about these facts. Those who have reservations are under no obligation to accept neurological criteria should they consider donating organs after death.

They are free to stipulate that death should be confirmed solely by the more traditional cardiopulmonary criteria. The fact that something is valid in principle does not mean that it is always wise or appropriate in practice. Circumstances may vary considerably.

But if human beings are, as the Church teaches, a union of intellective soul and material body, then death is rightly understood as the separation of the intellective soul from the body. This event would correspond with a complete cessation of all mental function. The cardiopulmonary standard, in fact, is just another means of determining brain death, for when heartbeat and respiration cease, the brain is deprived of oxygen. Within a few minutes, all brain function ceases. This is why it is so important, under the cardiopulmonary criteria, for physicians not to declare death until five minutes have passed. The brain has not yet lost its function, thus indicating that the soul has not yet departed. What medical science has shown us is that the cessation of brain function is the true sign of death.

All parties to the debate should realize that the use of neurological criteria is acceptable under Catholic teaching. That has been firmly decided. Patients, family members, and physicians are free to make use of these criteria as long as they are properly applied. Brain-death criteria ought to be standardized throughout the medical community and rigorously applied. Mistakes are sometimes made by physicians who declare a patient brain dead only to discover later on that they have revived. Even one such error is unacceptable and rightly causes widespread concern.

Waiting Lists and Xenotransplantation

There are not a sufficient number of organs for those in need of transplantation. The imbalance between need and availability can lead some to take desperate measures, as we saw above in the case of organ sales. Those without moral scruples who are able to buy organs will do so on the world market in an effort to preserve or extend their lives. A similar injustice occurs when those with wealth or personal connections use their power to increase their chances of moving up the waiting list. John Paul II, in his 2000 address to the Transplantation Society, notes that the only just means of distributing desperately needed organs is on the basis of "immunological and clinical factors."[9] Objective criteria must be the sole guide. Any distinctions drawn among persons based on personal characteristics, access to power, or the advantages of wealth is discriminatory. Every human being must be treated as an equal in God's sight.

One way to overcome the lack of transplantable human organs would be to use organs taken from animals. This is called xenotransplantation. The suggestion at first sounds fanciful or even offensive, but this is, in fact, a very promising avenue of research. The pig's heart, for example, is about the size of a human heart. If scientists could eliminate the possibility of any transmission of disease from pigs to humans, we would have an abundant supply of hearts for transplantation. The need for human donors would be greatly diminished, if not eliminated altogether. The Pontifical Academy for Life examines this possibility at length in its 2001 document, "Prospects for Xenotransplantation." [10]

Cloning, Human Embryos, and Stem Cells

In the final section of his 2000 address to the Transplantation Society, John Paul II expresses the hope of finding new methods of replacing failing organs, displaying the Catholic Church's longstanding support for progress in the sciences. He briefly mentions one promising scientific avenue: advanced prosthetics. The days of the wooden leg are far behind us. Prosthetics have achieved new levels of utility and natural function. Hip and knee replacements are routine. Recent evidence in animal models shows that the brain can exert direct control over artificial limbs through harmless brain implants. These facts open up whole new avenues for managing the loss of limbs and their functions.

For many years, the heart has been the subject of intense efforts to produce a mechanical replacement. Early artificial hearts, such as the Jarvik 7, managed to maintain the lives of patients for short periods of time and were often used as a stopgap until a donated organ became available. Devising a mechanical heart that will function as well as a natural one and that can serve as a permanent replacement for the human heart remains a challenging scientific goal.

The replacement hearts of the future may be grown in laboratories out of human tissue, using stem cells. There are various types of these cells, most of which do not raise any serious moral questions. Adult stem cells are plentiful and have many regenerative properties. We hear little about these successes. The media focuses its attention mainly on embryonic stem cells, which can be obtained only by destroying human embryos. John Paul II speaks out against "the manipulation and destruction of human embryos" in favor of "stem cells taken from adults."[11] This is the only morally appropriate course for the new and promising field of regenerative medicine.

At the time he gave his address, induced pluripotent stem cells had not yet been discovered. These cells are taken from born human beings and so begin as adult stem cells, but they are rendered pluripotent through a scientific process that enables them to return to an earlier undifferentiated state. The cells have a remarkable flexibility, which enables them to be redirected to various therapeutic purposes, such as the repair of damaged heart tissue. This flexibility is virtually identical to that found in human embryonic stem cells. So today we have an abundant source of stem cells with the same promising properties as human embryonic stem cells. These can be used not only in regenerative medicine, but also in efforts to grow artificial organs.

Donating an organ is a very serious decision. No one should approach it lightly. The Catholic Church provides an abundance of guidance on the proper means of donating organs, both while living and after death.

Notes

[1] John Paul II, Address to the Eighteenth International Congress of the Transplantation Society (August 29, 2000).

[2] Pius XII, Address to an International Congress of Anesthesiologists (November 24, 1957), reprinted in *National Catholic Bioethics Quarterly* 2.2 (Summer 2002): 309–314.

[3] John Paul II, Address to Transplantation Society, n. 2.

[4] Ibid, n. 4.

[5] Ibid.

[6] Ibid., n. 5.

[7] Ibid.

[8] Ibid.

[9] Ibid., n. 6, emphasis removed.

[10] Pontifical Academy for Life, *Prospects for Xenotransplantation: Scientific Aspects and Ethical Considerations* (September 26, 2001).

[11] John Paul II, Address to Transplantation Society, n. 8.

VI

STEM CELLS AND HUMAN DIGNITY

Marilyn E. Coors

A philanthropist who funds all types of stem cell research through a private family foundation remarked recently that the debate about human embryonic stem cell research is virtually settled in the scientific community; the only place it still rages is in the political arena. He was referring to a remarkable scientific breakthrough in stem cell technology called reprogrammed adult cells. This is the research of the future—and it is not implicated in the moral problems that plague human embryonic stem cell research. Yet large sums of money are still dedicated to human embryonic stem cell research in some states and private university foundations, and many politicians and even some scientists are adamantly committed to pursuing human embryonic stem cell research. The Catholic Church opposes human embryonic stem cell research because it involves the destruction of human embryos.[1]

This chapter will use human embryonic stem cell research as an example of a bioethical issue that embroils moral, scientific, and political components in a contentious public debate. The purpose is not to espouse a political position, but to discuss Catholic moral teaching about the dignity of human life with regard to human embryonic stem cell research and the pertinent scientific information. Debate over human embryonic stem cell research is illuminating, because it was the conviction of President George W. Bush's administration that precipitated the policy of limiting the use of federal funds for human embryonic stem cell research to a number of preexisting cell lines and increasing funding for adult stem cell research, a policy that was reversed by President Barack Obama's administration in 2009. Bush's funding structure provided a motivation, at least in part, for scientists to aggressively pursue the development of adult stem cell research, the reprogramming of adult cells, and other scientific technologies that avoid the ethical and moral issues surrounding the destruction of human embryos.

Consequently, morally acceptable advances in adult stem cell research have expanded dramatically, and the future holds many potential benefits for patients. It is possible that the future of stem cell research would look very different without powerful individuals at the highest level of government who were able to put federal funding at the service of morality.

Catholic Teaching on the Dignity of Life

The Catholic position on the dignity of human life as created in the image and likeness of God is the root of the Church's opposition to human embryonic stem cell research. *Donum vitae* provides the fundamental criterion on which the evaluation of all moral questions involving the human embryo rest:

> Thus the fruit of human generation, from the first moment of its existence, that is to say, from the moment the zygote has formed, demands the unconditional respect that is morally due to the human being in his bodily and spiritual totality. The human being is to be respected and treated as a person from the moment of conception; and therefore from that same moment his rights as a person must be recognized, among which in the first place is the inviolable right of every innocent human being to life.[2]

The teaching of *Donum vitae* is, in turn, grounded in Genesis: "Then God said, 'And now we will make human beings; they will be like us and resemble us'" (Gen. 1:26, GNV). One might logically ask how humans can resemble God since we have a mortal body made of flesh, while God is spirit? The traits that reflect God's likeness—to a greater or lesser degree—are our human intellect and free will. These differentiate us from all other species. Only human beings possess an intellect with which to think and reflect on the existence of God and enter into a relationship with him. He gives human beings these traits out of his extraordinary love for us. In addition, only human beings possess a free will to recognize good and evil and choose between them, the capacity of moral discernment. Even those persons who carry out evil acts are still capable of recognizing good by the use of their reason, and even though some persons choose evil, they remain capable of doing good through the exercise of their God-given free will.

The incarnation of Jesus through the virgin birth is a second moral reason why human beings deserve protection from the first moment of conception until natural death. When the angel Gabriel appeared to Mary and announced that the Holy Spirit would overshadow her and she would conceive and bear a child who would be the Son of God, the conception was supernatural (Luke 1:26–38). Yet the Bible tells us that the resulting pregnancy and birth were natural. Mary bore the child in her womb, and the Son of God took on flesh and came into the world like any other human baby. Jesus Christ was first an embryo, then a fetus, and then an infant, who was naked and vulnerable and in need of parents to nurture and protect him. The choice of God the Father to bring his Son into the world through the natural route of conception, gestation, and birth is the foundation for the dignity of humankind. Thus, the importance of human dignity as created in the image and likeness of God and the status of human beings as children of God through the Incarnation are extremely significant.

In contrast, if one departs from these theological underpinnings for the dignity of human life, as many secular philosophers, scientists, and others have, one must revert to the laborious identification of traits to define human dignity. Those traits could include language, cognition, reason, sense of personal identity, happiness, or sensitivity to pain, to name a few. Regardless of which cadre of traits one chooses to define human dignity, the distinction usually excludes those individuals among us who are disabled or cognitively impaired. Thus, it becomes readily apparent that once a society replaces the principle of the dignity of human life as created in the image of God with arbitrary traits, the result is hostility to any life that does not meet socially accepted standards.

The consequence of such a departure is apparent in human embryonic stem cell research, which justifies the use of embryos or fetuses by describing them as "just a clump of cells" that can be used as a tool of science. Actually, this statement is scientifically inaccurate, because every human embryo, given shelter and nourishment in a womb, will continue to develop as a human being, a feat that no other clump of cells is capable of! Moreover, future implications of this trend to devalue human life could potentially lead to the immoral use of nearly dead or newly dead human beings at the beginning or end of life for research.

Stem Cells

A recent instruction titled *Dignitas personae*, published by the Congregation for the Doctrine of the Faith and approved by Pope Benedict XVI in 2008, is relevant to this discussion. The purpose of *Dignitas personae* was to update *Donum vitae* (1987) regarding the great strides made by biomedical research in new possibilities for the treatment of disease and to address the serious questions these advances raise. *Dignitas personae* provides important guidance on the topic of stem cell research and other technologies. Before turning to this important document, let us briefly review the biology of stem cells, and why scientists are so excited about them.

Stem cells are undifferentiated or blank cells that exist in many parts of the human body, such as the bone marrow, circulating blood, umbilical cord blood, liver, gut, and pancreas. Cells from these sources are called adult stem cells, since they are found in tissues and organs in the adult body. Adult stem cells are fairly flexible in their ability to become many different types of cells that make up the human body. For example, bone marrow cells can be mobilized to become skin cells and heart cells. Because of this ability, adult stem cells have the potential to treat certain stem cell disorders such as leukemia, lymphoma, and autoimmune diseasesPotentially they may also be used to treat Parkinson's disease, liver disease, and others.

These types of cells, given their origins, do not violate the moral principles outlined above: "Methods which do not cause serious harm to the subject from whom the stem cells are taken are to be considered licit. This is generally the case when tissues are taken from: (a) an adult organism; (b) the blood of the umbilical cord at the time of birth; (c) fetuses who have died of natural causes."[3] Here are three sources of these promising cells, all readily available to the scientific community, which already provide cures for many serious diseases.

Adult stem cells also have the potential to repair or replace sections of organs. Currently, physicians in Europe have successfully transplanted a human windpipe using adult stem cells from the patient's own bone marrow to regenerate her damaged trachea following tuberculosis. Also promising are similar techniques to fashion bladders or regenerate skin with adult stem cells following burns. The hope is that treatments such as these will expand and improve. However, as with any medical procedure, there are risks involved in with adult stem cell treatment, such as rejection or infection, but the observed benefits far outweigh the risks. Adult stem cell treatments, such as bone marrow transplantation, have over a fifty-year history of treating over eighty disorders successfully, and the number is growing.

Another far more controversial source of stem cells is the early embryo; cells obtained from this source are called human embryonic stem cells. To obtain human embryonic stem cells, scientists destroy the embryo at about five days of life, when it consists of about a hundred and fifty to two hundred cells, and harvest the cells from the interior of the embryo. "The obtaining of stem cells from a living human embryo, on the other hand, invariably causes the death of the embryo and is consequently gravely illicit: 'research, in such cases, irrespective of efficacious therapeutic results, is not truly at the service of humanity.'"[4] The scientifically enticing aspects of human embryonic stem cells are threefold. First, human embryonic stem cells possess the ability to differentiate into *all* tissues and organs that make up the human body. Second, they hold the key to understanding the development and growth of human life in health and disease. Third, they may provide biological clues to aid discovery of the long-sought-after "fountain of youth."

The hope of scientists who work with these cells is that human embryonic stem cells, on their own, will be used to treat otherwise untreatable diseases. At the time of this writing, there were only two clinical trials involving human embryonic stem cell treatments approved by the Food and Drug Administration. In 2010, the Geron Corporation enrolled the first patient in a clinical trial using human embryonic stem cell treatment for severe thoracic spinal cord injury to assess safety and tolerability; the trial closed abruptly in 2012 because of insufficient funds. In 2011, Advanced Cell Technology initiated a clinical trial that uses human embryonic stem cells to treat patients with macular degeneration. The results of these trials will take years to assess. However, the potential for human embryonic stem cells to cure disease is far off at best and probably unlikely, regardless of what you read or hear in the media. The primary reason for this is that human embryonic stem cells are rejected by patients, and thus treatments that make use of them require the immunosuppression of recipients, which entails significant side effects. Another reason that the direct use of human embryonic stem cells is unlikely for clinical purposes is that studies have shown them to cause nonmalignant tumors in animals, raising serious questions about their safety in humans.

A second reason that human embryonic stem cells are interesting to scientists is that these cells may hold the key to understanding how human development unfolds in health and disease. This newfound knowledge could lead to the development of new drugs and other therapies. An example of a moral clinical procedure that is the result of understanding the biological process of human development but did not involve human embryonic stem cell research is fetal surgery to correct spina bifida prior to birth. When the surgery is successful, it greatly improves the health outcome for the child.

However, the use of knowledge of human development can also be immoral. An example of an immoral process would be the creation of a human embryo via in vitro fertilization whose intelligence had been intentionally diminished below what is considered normal for a member of our species. The purpose would be to produce human-like creatures with lesser intelligence to perform dangerous and undesirable tasks for society; this procedure would be immoral both in intent and in action. It is not yet possible to design beings with diminished intelligence, but human degradation is one of the implications of biomedical research that concerned Pope St. John Paul II, based on the potential for genetic manipulation.[5]

There is a third aspect of human embryonic stem cell research that is not discussed much, but it is one that may be important in the minds of some scientists, though these comments are speculative at this time. One of the properties that define human embryonic stem cells is "immortality": they have the ability to remain in culture in an undifferentiated state virtually forever. When scientists understand the genetic factors that give rise to this "immortality" and the gene products that make it possible, scientists could be on the path to discovering the "fountain of youth." Just imagine the power, fame, and fortune involved if such a discovery occurs! For example, there is evidence in our culture of a tremendous demand among aging baby boomers for existing products with the potential to enhance capabilities (e.g., Ritalin for increased "focus," cosmetic surgery) or lengthen life (health food fads and dietary supplements). This consumer demand provides some evidence that a genetic alternative to prevent aging would garner great interest. While the mere attempt to extend the human lifespan is not immoral in itself, it certainly would entail significant social, financial, and other existential challenges, not to mention the contradiction of the Catholic belief that our eternal life is not meant for this world but in heaven with God.

Despite the potential for abuse, understanding the aging process at the molecular level could lead to treatment of the devastating childhood disease known as Hutchinson-Gilford progeria syndrome, an accelerated aging disease that affects children. The identification of the genetic basis of HGPS led scientists to the experimental drug that is in clinical trials at the time of this writing. This is the first step in solving the tragic puzzle of HGPS for the children and families who suffer with this disease. It is important to remember that the pursuit of knowledge is good and endorsed by Church teaching; only the abuse of knowledge is immoral. The magisterium encourages the pursuit of science as an *"invaluable service to the integral good of the life and dignity of every human being."*[6]

Exploitation of Women

In his 1995 letter to women, John Paul II observes that women have been the subjects of exploitation and violence throughout time. He denounces all forms of exploitation of women:

> When it comes to setting women free from every kind of exploitation and domination, the Gospel contains an ever relevant message which goes back to the attitude of Jesus Christ himself. Transcending the established norms of his own culture, Jesus treated women with openness, respect, acceptance and tenderness. In this way he honoured the dignity which women have always possessed according to God's plan and in his love.[7]

A new form of exploitation of women exists in the realm of human embryonic stem cell research and some fertility treatments. This is the recruitment of young women to provide eggs in return for financial reimbursement. When the need for embryos for stem cell research and some infertility treatments exceeds the supply from in vitro fertilization clinics, scientists recruit young women to provide their eggs for compensation. This is usually accomplished by harvesting eggs through a procedure that includes hyperstimulation of the ovaries with potent drugs followed by the surgical harvesting of the eggs.

The payment for women undergoing this "inconvenience" is from five thousand to ten thousand dollars. If the eggs are destined to be used to treat another woman's infertility, the payment can reach as high as a hundred thousand dollars for highly desirable eggs. Desirable eggs are typically those of women who are tall, athletic, smart, and attractive according to societal standards.

The physical risks of egg harvesting range from general discomfort to clotting and stroke; psychological risks have not been documented. The physical risks are obviously significant, and the procedure also includes serious moral issues and justice implications.

According to Catholic teaching, it is immoral to provide eggs for any purpose, just as it is immoral to produce a human embryo only to destroy it for research or to treat the infertility of another woman.[8] Moreover, egg harvesting is also unjust because it targets young women in need of financial resources, for example students or underprivileged women. The compensation for eggs offers incentives to women in need of resources that could skew their evaluation of the morality and physical risks of the procedure and compromise the voluntariness of their decision to participate. The injustice involved in payment for eggs is exacerbated in challenging economic times.

An article in the *Wall Street Journal* in February 2009 reported an increase in the numbers of egg donors among educated women who needed to pay mounting tuition bills and among underprivileged women who needed to pay bills.[9] Women who are not in need of funds would typically not undertake the risks of this procedure merely to advance science. This has been documented in countries like England, where compensation for eggs was illegal, with the exception of reimbursement for transportation and other minor costs. Egg donation in the absence of compensation resulted in an insufficient supply of eggs for research and infertility treatments, causing the legal restriction against compensation for eggs to be lifted in England in 2010. This practice of providing eggs for research constitutes another important moral concern that undergirds the Church's objection to human embryonic stem cell research.

Reprogrammed (Induced Pluripotent) Stem Cells

Recently, scientists have discovered a way to reprogram adult skin and other body cells into embryonic-like stem cells called induced pluripotent stem cells (iPSCs). This does not involve the use of embryos or their destruction. These iPSCs are made in the laboratory by introducing a mixture of genes to developed adult cells to return (or reprogram) them to an undeveloped state.[10] The combination of genes works to reverse the wiring of the genome of adult cells and turns back the clock to when the cells were still in their embryonic state, making them pluripotent. Pluripotent means that cells can produce many tissues in the human body. The gold standard test for pluripotency is the ability of a cell to change into all cell types. The iPSCs created by reprogramming pass this test. The second criterion that distinguishes pluripotent stem cells is the formation of nonmalignant tumors that contain many different kinds of cells called teratomas, and iPSCs pass this test as well. These two traits demonstrate that reprogramming can produce iPSCs that behave like embryonic stem cells with subtle differences.

At the time of this writing, the hope of clinical use of iPSC therapies to treat diseases in humans is still futuristic, but two groundbreaking studies in animal models provide the proof of principle that the hope might one day be realized.[11] First, the transplantation of iPSCs into mice affected with the sickle-cell anemia gene saw the iPSCs integrated stably and the disease corrected. Second, iPSCs introduced into the brain of a rat model of Parkinson's disease implanted and resulted in functional recovery.

These advances in iPSCs are very encouraging because they provide evidence of the value of iPSCs as a model with which to study disease mechanisms, discover new therapies, and develop personalized treatments without immunosuppression or the destruction of human embryos. The safety issues involved with iPSCs are not yet resolved, and these crucial challenges must be overcome for iPSCs to realize their full potential.

Unconditional Respect for Human Life

The fundamental principle that grounds the Church's teaching regarding these technologies is the unconditional respect for all human life from the moment of conception until natural death. The dignity of the human person mandates that the life of one person should never be sacrificed to save the life of another. Consequently, if a biomedical technique manipulates human life for immoral purposes, uses life as a tool of research, or measures the value of a human life by a yardstick based on socially defined acceptable traits, it is immoral.

Dignitas personae expresses a great yes to the inalienable value and dignity of every human life and supports the "invaluable service" of scientific research when it attempts to cure disease or restore normal human function through moral means. It also calls Catholic lay persons and medical professionals to understand the reasons that underscore the Church's teaching and to take action to defend the vulnerable condition of human embryos in order to promote a more humane civilization.

Notes

1 See Congregation for the Doctrine of the Faith, *Donum vitae* (February 27, 1987), II.1; and CDF, *Dignitas personae* (September 8, 2008), n. 12.

2 CDF, *Donum vitae*, I.1.

3 CDF, *Dignitas personae*, n. 32.

4 Ibid.

5 John Paul II, "Address on Medical Ethics and Genetic Manipulation," *Origins* 13.23 (November 17, 1983): 386–389.

6 CDF, *Dignitas personae*, n. 3, original emphasis.

7 John Paul II, Letter to Women (June 29, 1995), n. 3.

8 CDF, *Donum vitae*, II.2.

9 Bari Weiss, "Putting Herself on Sale," *Wall Street Journal*, February 6, 2009.

10 Jane Rossant, "Stem Cells: The Magic Brew," *Nature* 448.7151 (July 19, 2007): 260–262.

11 Daisy A. Robinton and George Q. Daley, "The Promise of Induced Pluripotent Stem Cells in Research and Therapy," *Nature* 481.7381 (January 18, 2012): 295–305.

VII

GENETIC SCREENING, TESTING, AND ENGINEERING

Marilyn E. Coors

In 2003, scientists completed deciphering the human genome and launched the world into an unprecedented era of biotechnology and genetic medicine. Catholics experience genetic medicine predominantly through testing to diagnose the cause of disease or disability affecting themselves or their families. Genetic testing is offered in the doctor's office or, increasingly, through direct-to-consumer testing from companies. The influence of genetic medicine will only continue to expand in coming years. For this reason, Catholics should understand the promises and perils that could accompany new genetic discoveries: there may be moments when you are called on to decide whether or not to use a new medical procedure for yourselves or your loved ones; or you may have opportunities to support or reject new procedures publicly or in the voting booth.

The Catholic Church is not anti-genetics, as some would like to believe. The Church supports science; in fact, Pope Francis is the first pontiff with a scientific background. Prior to entering the seminary and studying philosophy and theology, he trained as a chemical technician and received a master's degree in chemistry. His background is an important asset in engaging scientists in thought-provoking and constructive discussions concerning advances in genetics, as previous popes have done. Moreover, the Congregation for the Doctrine of the Faith has affirmed that "the Magisterium also seeks to offer a word of support and encouragement for the perspective on culture which considers science an invaluable service to the integral good of the life and dignity of every human being."[1]

In addition, the 2009 conference sponsored by the Pontifical Academy for Life, titled "New Frontiers of Genetics and the Risk of Eugenics," highlighted the significance of the advances in genetics and praised recent breakthroughs, but also warned that "excesses can 'lead to so-called eugenics, which, in its various forms, seeks to obtain the perfect human being,' which includes unethical means that violate respect of all forms and conditions of human life."[2] At the conference, Bishop Rino Fisichella, then-President of the Pontifical Academy for Life, stated that it would be a mistake to think that the idea of eugenics has vanished, just because it remains unpopular to openly promote it. The concerns that the conference addressed are real, and the future will only see an increase in the potentially beneficial and harmful uses of new genetic discoveries.

Moving forward, we will consider the scientific and moral aspects of genetic screening and testing and genetic engineering, including the ways in which these technologies can be used for moral or immoral purposes. The analysis hinges on standards articulated in *Dignitas personae*, which states that scientific advances are moral when they serve to cure diseases and reestablish the normal functioning of persons.[3] Scientific advances are immoral and cannot be utilized when they involve the destruction of human beings, when they include means that contradict the dignity of the person, or when they are used for purposes contrary to the integral good of humankind.

Genetic Screening and Testing

Many reports differentiate between genetic testing and genetic screening, while others use the terms interchangeably. Genetic testing directly analyzes the DNA or chromosomes to determine the status of individuals who are at risk for a particular inherited condition. Genetic screening uses the same type of DNA analysis, but instead analyzes a target population in which early detection may help to avoid the consequences of a disease. In this sense, genetic screenings are useful for both prenatal diagnosis and for detecting rare metabolic diseases in newborns such as phenylketonuria (a disease that causes intellectual disability and can be prevented by following a special diet), sickle cell anemia, and Tay-Sachs disease in Ashkenazi Jews.

Screening is also useful to identify individuals that are carriers of a chromosome abnormality or a gene that may cause problems for either the person screened or their offspring. The purpose of predictive genetic screening is to benefit the individual tested, and the screening test should have sufficient clinical value to justify its use.

The Morality of Prenatal Genetic Screening and Testing

Medicine is rapidly becoming more technical. Consequently, doctors often expect patients to understand complex facts to make informed health care choices for themselves and their loved ones. This is particularly true in the area of prenatal genetic screening, which is routine in obstetrical practice to detect genetic changes associated with disease or disability. It is currently recommended that all pregnant women undergo a screening for Down syndrome, neural tube defects, and other genetic disorders (such as trisomy 18). Certain prenatal genetic screenings may be required by law on a state-by-state basis, and an ever-increasing number of other genetic tests are optional at this time. Prenatal genetic screening can pose questions of risk, hope, heartbreak, and conscience to parents who are faced with decisions about which procedures to undergo.

Prenatal genetic screening underwent a revolution in 2010 with the introduction of a noninvasive test that can detect genetic abnormalities by isolating and analyzing fetal DNA in the mother's blood.[4] This was a departure from previous screening methods that relied on ultrasound markers and levels of blood chemicals to predict the genetic status of a fetus; only follow-up invasive tests like amniocentesis or chorionic villus sampling that entail the risk of miscarriage could diagnose a genetic abnormality in the fetus. This has now changed. The noninvasive prenatal diagnosis can potentially test for hundreds or thousands of genetic abnormalities, from heart defects and leukemia to a range of disorders involving impairment of mental function. Moreover, parents can have the entire genome of a fetus sequenced and learn about all of its genes prior to birth.

These new procedures are a sea change in prenatal diagnosis and could become the choice of parents who want the maximum amount of information about their fetus. However, expanded testing raises the concern that the results will increase abortions and confuse or alarm many couples. Critics say that some tests have not been thoroughly validated and can produce misleading results or have low clinical utility, which could lead to unnecessary anxiety.[5] The positive aspect of these new tests is that some can identify disorders early and potentially benefit the fetus. There are a number of moral uses of prenatal testing. For example, testing is moral when its purpose is to treat or heal the fetus through therapeutic interventions.[6] Another moral use of prenatal testing is to provide parents with information and assistance in making decisions about a course of action that is beneficial to the fetus. Those decisions could include choice of hospital, mode of delivery, emotional and psychological preparation for the birth of a child with special needs, and interventions to improve the health of the fetus.

According to Catholic teaching, prenatal testing is immoral when results indicating an abnormality lead to a decision to abort a fetus with a genetic disorder, disability, or predisposition to disease. For example, it is reported that there is a 60 to 90 percent rate of termination of pregnancies following a Down syndrome diagnosis; notably, Hispanic women are less likely to terminate a pregnancy after diagnosis of Down syndrome.[7] In contemporary society, the social expectation following a diagnosis of Down syndrome is termination of the pregnancy. In some instances, the expectation escalates to a sense of obligation to "do something"—meaning to abort the fetus because of the disorder. However, that expectation may be changing somewhat as families have more support for children with Down syndrome, who are now integrated into mainstream education.

Going against the current, the Church teaches that, contrary to some social expectations, it is immoral for parents to pursue—or worse yet, for society to dictate—the use of prenatal testing for eugenic purposes to eliminate gene-based disabilities or undesirable traits through abortion, or by selecting only certain embryos for implantation because of the notion that certain types of lives are not worth living. In 2009, Pope Benedict XVI spoke out against the "obsessive search for the perfect child."[8] He indicated his concern that "a new mentality is creeping in that tends to justify a different consideration of life and personal dignity."[9] In 2010, before he became Pope, Francis echoed this position in more scientific terms in his defense of the right to life for the unborn: "The moral problem of abortion is pre-religious in nature because the genetic code of the person happens in the moment of conception. ... A human being is already there. I separate the topic of abortion from any religious concept. It is a scientific problem. ... To not let the development continue of a being who already has all the genetic code of a human being is not ethical."[10]

The trend to eliminate children with genetic defects is disturbing on a second, related front. As the number of people living with disabilities decreases, it becomes more likely that those who do live with disabilities will experience negative labeling and discrimination. The federal Genetic Information Nondiscrimination Act prohibits discrimination based on genetic information.[11] However, it is a matter of human psychology that attitudes change along with changes in technology. Proponents of selective abortion increasingly argue that the abortion of undesirable fetuses is not discrimination but a merciful act performed to prevent these children from suffering and to prevent society from bearing the associated financial costs. Pressure for selective abortion is already exerted by some medical professionals, insurance companies, friends, and relatives, and the pressure is not likely to abate.

Many people living with genetic disabilities rightly challenge the predominant social narrative, for they see new genetic discoveries as threats of annihilation for persons like themselves.[12] Francis demonstrated the depth of Christ's love for persons with disabilities when he halted a weekly audience in 2013 to kiss and hold a disfigured believer with neurofibromatosis, a rare genetic disease that causes growths covering the body, impaired vision, and in some cases cancer. Patients suffering from neurofibromatosis are often shunned by society because of their appearance. The Church teaches that all human beings possess inherent dignity and the right to life because they are created in the image of God. Parents thus have an obligation to accept and love their children unconditionally as God does—just as they are. The Catholic ideal is that parents welcome their newborn child without reservation rather than judging the child's fitness as a condition of their love and acceptance. The Catholic notion of human well-being celebrates diversity, and the Church teaches that parental love should strive to exemplify the love of Christ for his Church, despite the imperfections, disappointments, and anguish that always accompany parenting.

What Can Genetic Testing Really Tell Us?

There is a growing concern that genetic testing could be used to detect a rapidly expanding list of genetic variations that indicate an increased risk, not a diagnosis, for common complex diseases like cancer, diabetes (type 2), mental illness, and other conditions, some of which do not manifest until adulthood. In the future, it is possible that similar tests could identify predispositions to such traits as obesity, addiction, sexual orientation, or specific behaviors. Test results for traits and behaviors are ambiguous at best, since such results indicate only predisposition, not causation. For example, a positive result could indicate that a baby has a fifty-fifty chance of expressing a particular trait just 1 to 5 percent of the time, which means the result has little or no predictive value.

Genetics and Homosexuality

Since the topic of homosexuality is so sensitive and high profile in our religious, political, and legal debates, let us analyze it as an example of what genetic testing can and cannot tell us about human behavior. Behaviors like homosexuality are thought to result from the complex interactions of many genes, plus environment and will. There is a long-standing debate about the role of genetic factors influencing homosexual behavior. The debate usually poses the following question: are people homosexual by nature or are they homosexual by choice? Translated, that means is there a gene that causes homosexuality, or is it merely a personal preference?

Science at the present time has not identified a gene associated with homosexual behavior, because reports of a gene related to homosexual behavior have not been replicated, which is the gold standard for scientific research.[13] A 2000 study reports that genetic factors may play a role in homosexual behavior (i.e., identical twins are both more likely to practice homosexual behavior than fraternal twins or fraternal twins and their non-twin siblings) along with environmental influences like parents, friends, media, and popular culture.[14] The results of the study are weakened by the small numbers of participants and low statistical power.[14]

Even if future research identifies a gene associated with homosexuality, that gene will not dictate human behavior in a cause-and-effect way, because human behavior is complex. We know this from other traits such as addiction and obesity; behavioral traits are influenced by the cumulative interplay of many genes contributing small effects, with environment and will playing important roles. Because we are beings endowed with reason and free will by God, behavior will always encompass an act of will that involves a decision to pursue one action and reject another. It is extremely difficult for persons with a predisposition to homosexuality or substance abuse to resist that behavior, and it may be impossible without God's grace, but we have a loving God who has promised to give us the grace to live according to his teachings.

The *Catechism of the Catholic Church* teaches that homosexual persons "must be accepted with respect, compassion, and sensitivity. Every sign of unjust discrimination in their regard should be avoided."[15] Francis referred to this teaching in a 2013 press interview: "If a person is gay and seeks the Lord and has good will, well who am I to judge them? The Catechism explains this in a very beautiful way. ... It says these persons must not be marginalized for this; they must be integrated into society."[16] Francis is calling those whose particular temptation is same-sex attraction to seek God by living for and obeying the teachings of Christ, and he calls the Church to encourage and not condemn these persons.

Human Genetic Engineering

Human genetic engineering means the technological modification of human genes. Its purpose is twofold: (1) healing of disease through gene therapy by transferring a copy of a normal functioning gene into the cells of a patient who possesses a malfunctioning copy; and (2) enhancement above what is normal function by modifying the genetic makeup of an otherwise healthy person. Genetic engineering is no longer limited to science fiction; it is now a common focus in clinical trials and research. Moreover, from the huge demands for designer drugs, cosmetic surgery, and diet and exercise regiments promising human perfection, it seems likely that there will be a ready market for genetic engineering if it becomes safe and effective. It is important that we comprehend this distinction between therapy and enhancement to understand the Church's teaching and apply it to the moral assessment of new genetic developments.

Pope St. John Paul II discussed the morality of biotechnology use in an address to the World Medical Association at the Vatican in 1983.[17] He implicitly endorsed biotechnology and invited participation in the work of the Creator through progress in genetics: "The researcher follows God's design. God willed man to be the king of creation." John Paul II supported genetic engineering that is therapeutic and aimed at healing disease and stated that it "will be considered in principle as desirable, provided that it tends to real promotion of the personal well-being of man, without harming his integrity or worsening his life conditions." He offered a caution about genetic engineering that goes beyond the strictly therapeutic and enters the realm of enhancement, emphasizing the importance of morally analyzing each new advance, but he was optimistically open to new developments: "It is really of great interest to know whether an intervention upon the genetic store, exceeding the bounds of the therapeutic in the strict sense, is morally acceptable as well." The Church holds that any genetic manipulation that is moral should truly improve the human condition for some persons without worsening the lives of others.[18]

Recently, Archbishop Gianfranco Girotti, in an interview titled "The New Forms of Social Sin," told the Vatican newspaper, *L'Osservatore Romano*, that the largely uncharted work of bioethics is a great danger zone for the modern soul. He stated that within bioethics "we cannot deny the existence of violations of fundamental rights of human nature—this occurs by way of experiments and genetic modifications, whose results we cannot easily predict or control."[19]

Once genetic engineering is directed at improving the human biological condition rather than correcting defects, the manipulation entails greater moral significance. Some of the questions that should be considered in the moral analysis of genetic engineering include, What would truly constitute an improvement (resistance to disease, better memory, higher intelligence, greater strength, lower sleep requirement)? Who would decide? Would the change be available to all? and Will the change be a real improvement in a future time or in another culture, since genetic changes are most likely permanent? Most of the important questions surrounding genetic manipulation are extremely complicated, requiring deliberate and careful moral analysis and time to carefully assess the scientific results of preliminary animal studies.

As science progresses, the technologies will change and the Church will assess each procedure individually and collectively. The Church has always provided insightful and well-informed guidance for her members and will continue to do so. For example, John Paul II outlined several timeless conditions that must be met for genetic interventions to be moral.[20] First, the biological integrity of every human being as a unity composed of body and soul must be respected. Second, embryonic life must be accorded the basic rights that all humans deserve. Finally, alteration of the genome may not aim at the creation of new or different groups of people. These truths are constant measures of morality in the midst of rapidly changing technology. It is theoretically possible that genetic engineering could be truly beneficial for individuals and society and at the same time respect the dignity of the person, but the present state of the science generally does not meet this requirement.

Respecting the Dignity of the Human Person

As far back as 1983, John Paul II expressed concern that genetic testing and manipulation could result in differences that "provoke fresh marginalization" in our world by enhancing or diminishing human traits. He was concerned that genetic manipulation could actually dehumanize the human person through an over emphasis on genes and a lack of respect for the dignity of every person as created in the image of God. Dehumanization tends to reify the genome as the most important element of being human, ignoring the impact of God, human spirit, environment, cultural origins, faith, and human dignity. The more science learns about the human genome, the more we are tempted to explain everything in terms of genetics. While we certainly can understand human beings in part by our genetic makeup, we are much more than the sum of our genes. Rather, human dignity is an inherent property of the person as created in the image of God, and dignity is not dependent on possession of a list of traits or characteristics (language, rationality, etc.).

In Genesis, God gives humans the mandate to be stewards of creation with the limitation that humans should not eat of the tree of good and evil. Therein lies the concern. The idea that the human mind—with our newfound and modest understanding of genetics—could design real and safe improvements to the human being is likely mere hubris. The complexity and interdependence of the human genome is difficult to understand and even more difficult to manipulate safely. Our impending power to alter our genetic heritage, coupled with a limited ability to predict the consequences of those alterations, cries out for a cautious and humble approach to new genetic discoveries.

For Reflection

God is the Creator and originator of human life; only He fully understands how "fearfully and wonderfully" we are made (Ps. 139:14).

Notes

[1] Congregation for the Doctrine of the Faith (CDF), *Dignitas personae* (September 8, 2008), n. 3.

[2] "Economic Interests Drive Wider Acceptance of Eugenics, Says Archbishop," *Catholic News and Herald*, February 20, 2009.

[3] CDF, *Dignitas personae*, n. 4.

[4] Henry T. Greeley, "Get Ready for the Flood of Fetal Gene Screening," *Nature* 469.7330 (January 20, 2011): 289–291.

[5] Cecile Muller and Linda D. Cameron, "Trait Anxiety, Information Modality, and Responses to Communications about Prenatal Genetic Testing," *Journal of Behavioral Medicine* 37.5 (October 2014): 988–999.

[6] Elio Cardinal Sgreccia, "Ethical Issues in Prenatal Diagnosis and Fetal Therapy: A Catholic Perspective," *Fetal Therapy* 4.suppl (1989): 19–27.

[7] Jamie J. Natoli, "Prenatal Diagnosis of Down Syndrome: A Systematic Review of Termination Rates," *Prenatal Diagnosis* 32.2 (February 2012): 142–153.

[8] John Thavis, "Pope Denounces Trend toward 'Designer Babies,'" *Catholic News Service*, February 26, 2007.

[9] Gina Salamone, "Custom-Made Babies Delivered: Fertility Clinic Doctor's Design-A-Kid Offer Creates Uproar," *New York Daily News*, March 4, 2009.

[10] Jimmy Akin, "Pope Francis on Abortions and Homosexual 'Marriage,'" *Catholic Answers*, April 13, 2013, reviewing *On Heaven and Earth: On Faith, Family and the Church in the 21st Century*, by Jorge Mario Bergoglio and Abraham Skorka (New York: Random House, 2010).

[11] Genetic Information Nondiscrimination Act of 2008, Pub. L. No. 110–233, 122 Stat. 881 (2008).

[12] Ellen Painter Dollar, "Messy Stories: Disabilities and the Choices Parents Make," *Christian Century* 130.23 (November 13, 2013), http://www.christiancentury.org/.

[13] Vincent Savolainen and Laurent Lehmann, "Evolutionary Biology: Genetics and Bisexuality," *Nature* 445.7124 (January 11, 2007): 158–159.

[14] Kenneth S. Kendler et al., "Sexual Orientation in a U.S. National Sample of Twin and Nontwin Sibling Pairs," *American Journal of Psychiatry* 157.11 (November 1, 2000): 1843–1846.

[15] *Catechism*, n. 2358.

[16] "Pope Francis: In His Own Words—Selected Quotes from the First Year of Francis's Pontificate," *Catholic Herald*, March 13, 2014.

[17] John Paul II, Address on Medical Ethics and Genetic Manipulation, *Origins* 13.23 (November 17, 1983), n. 6.

[18] Albert S. Moraczewski and John B. Shea, "Genetic Medicine," in *Catholic Health Care Ethics: A Manual*

for Practitioners, ed. Edward J. Furton, Peter J. Cataldo, and Albert S. Moraczewski (Philadelphia: National Catholic Bioethics Center, 2009), 241.

[19] Gianfranco Girotti, quoted in Nicola Gori, "The New Forms of Social Sin," *L'Osservatore Romano*, March 9, 2008.

[20] John Paul II, Address on Medical Ethics and Genetic Manipulation.

VIII

End-of-Life Issues

Archbishop José H. Gomez

Our culture tries to avoid the topic: Newspapers shun the words "death" and "dying," using words like "passing away" or "deceased" instead. Action movies avoid the fear and mystery of death by turning it into an entertaining part of a fantasy to eliminate the bad guys. Many people desperately turn to medicine to avoid death and prolong life at all costs. Others, when facing the lingering death of a relative, may wish to relieve their loved one's misery by "putting him to sleep," as a veterinarian would a dying pet.

The Christian Meaning of Death

God created man for immortality (Wisd. 2:23–24), but now—with Adam's sin—pain, suffering, and death mark our earthly existence (Rom. 5:12–14). Death should not paralyze us with fear but should help us appreciate the meaning of our Christian lives, motivating us to overcome our sinfulness, be reconciled to God, and live our lives in the service of God and others. Let us remember that Christ conquered death by freely dying on the cross and rising again. Jesus redeems death, transforming it into the door to eternal life with him and with our redeemed loved ones.

For Christians, the process of dying is a wonderful purification from attachments to sensual pleasures that prepares us to desire the only object worthy of our love: God. By respecting God's dominion over life and death, we facilitate his work with souls—their potential conversion and that of their relatives—and prepare them for their definitive communion with God in heaven.

End-of-Life Dilemmas

A few years ago, we witnessed with horror the death of Terri Schindler Schiavo, a defenseless woman in a persistent vegetative state. Her parents and siblings accompanied Terri in her last agonizing hours, unable to do anything to prevent her agony because the state had mandated her "death with dignity" by means of dehydration. This aroused much debate over the meaning of life and of a dignified death, a legitimate debate in which the Catholic Church participates. The terms of the debate have changed, however, now that scientific advances make it possible to prolong or destroy human life in unimaginable ways: we can now keep the heart, lungs, and other body parts going almost indefinitely. But is this what God wants for us? In using such measures, do we not treat people almost like machines?

We hate to see the suffering of loved ones unnecessarily prolonged by life support. We know they will die soon, and maybe we are asking ourselves, Can't we end their ordeal by "pulling the plug" or allowing the nurse to administer a sedative? Would this be murder? Does it respect the God-given dignity of the human person and God's dominion over life and death?

Considering my own life and possible future illnesses and medical needs, can I avoid burdening my family and loved ones with situations in which they feel compelled to keep me alive at all costs? Can I make a "living will" prohibiting certain extraordinary treatments? Can I request that certain treatments be terminated if I become "brain dead"? Would such a request be equivalent to suicide?

What if a person's life becomes "worthless," and he becomes a mindless "vegetable"? Are we required to keep him alive? What if he was a drug addict? Should we waste valuable medical resources to keep an irresponsible drug addict alive?

Other questions might arise over transplantation. If it would be useful, a person might want to offer organs for transplantation. But what if doctors require removing a key vital organ like the heart before bodily disintegration begins? Is there any risk that removing those organs too soon constitutes the taking of life? When would it be morally permissible for doctors to remove unpaired vital organs? Are there instructions I should give for the use of my organs?

Life Is a Gift from God

God creates us in his image and likeness, sharing with us the sacred gift of life that enables us to act freely. He calls us to the fullness of a life of love as his children (Eph. 1:3–4 and John 1:10–12), into loving communion with him. Human life thus is and remains sacred forever. We should continue to respect and care for his gift by using reasonable means of preserving our lives, such as proper nourishment, rest, and health care.

For Christians, death does not end life but moves it to a new stage. Although we naturally fear death, a person with faith believes that death is the beginning of a definitive encounter with God in heaven and the marvelous fulfillment of life. So we should never treat this gift as absolute: to hang onto life at all costs implies that we do not want to be with God, that we love the gift (of life) more than the One who gives it.

Euthanasia

In contrast to our understanding of life and death, there is a popular view of euthanasia as so-called death with dignity. *Euthanasia* comes from the Greek *eu* (meaning "beautiful" or "good") and *thanatos* ("death"). The common understanding of euthanasia—*a good or beautiful death*—is the death of another person caused intentionally to eliminate suffering.[1]

Euthanasia has other meanings, often leading to contradictory ideas. Some use it to refer to the elimination of people whose lives are considered "unworthy" because of handicap, illness, or old age—a practice that is always wrong. Others use it to describe pain control in terminally ill patients or the voluntary refusal of useless or disproportionate therapies—practices that are often reasonable and acceptable. But one word cannot be used to describe moral opposites without causing great confusion.

Euthanasia eliminates not only the suffering of a person but also the person who suffers.

God is the Lord of life and death; usurping God's dominion by deliberately killing a human being makes euthanasia murder. The Church thus condemns all forms of euthanasia, whether they are accomplished by *passive* omissions (intentionally denying patients reasonable and necessary treatments) or by *active* means, such as the injection of lethal drugs, and whether they are *voluntary* (requested by the patient) or *involuntary* (without the patient's request or consent).

Death with Dignity

Some think legalizing euthanasia would give the terminally ill the right to die "with dignity." This presumes that suffering is "undignified." Suffering is truly distressing, but it does not take away our human dignity. In contrast, killing persons who are terminally ill does take away their dignity, since it says implicitly that they are not human or worthy of life. Under the guise of doing good ("mercy killing"), legalized euthanasia has historically led to barbaric abuses. The Nazis, for example, began by euthanizing very young children who were sick or disabled, then moved to older children and adults who were terminally ill, had Down syndrome, or had other physical or mental limitations.

Death is *dignified* when the essential dignity of the human person is respected throughout the dying process. This means ending one's existence according to God's plan, without human hastening. It recognizes that our existence comes from God and that He calls us to himself at the end. It allows a person to die, so far as possible, in possession of his faculties, comforted by loved ones and aided by the spiritual and sacramental gifts of our faith. To help a patient die with dignity, the Church offers the sacraments of Anointing of the Sick, Confession, and Holy Communion, accompanied by our prayers.

Life and Consciousness

A serious accident or illness may leave a person in a coma or persistent vegetative state. Such a person is unconscious and unable to communicate. Some see in such a state a lack of human intelligence or free will. Consequently, some consider individuals in a coma or persistent vegetative state to be non-persons.

But God creates all human beings in his image and likeness, integrally coupling our human and spiritual existence. We never lose this likeness. To think otherwise is to condition our dignity as children of God on external manifestations of intelligence and freedom. If those in a coma are not human, we would have to conclude that people who are sleeping or intoxicated are also not human, since they too are unable to manifest their humanity. If that were true and one were to kill another person while he slept, one would not really have murdered a person—an obviously absurd statement. Being unconscious and incapable of communicating does not mean that one is not free and rational; it only means that the normal expression of those attributes is inactive.

A person who appears to be unconscious may actually feel pain, hear, and remember experiences. In 1995, for example, Kate Adamson had a rare double brain-stem stroke at the age of thirty-three. She was completely paralyzed for seventy days and was unable to move or speak, but she could hear. She heard the medical staff make plans to remove her feeding tube and starve her to death, and she had no nourishment for eight days, but she recovered: "I could feel everything the doctors did to me, and I could do nothing. I was at the complete mercy of others, and they couldn't hear me." [2]

Countless people have recovered from the so-called persistent vegetative state—a state lasting more than a year in which a person shows no response to stimuli. Medicine still cannot accurately diagnose which patients will or will not recover from this condition.

It is important that we treat those in a coma or persistent vegetative state as human persons. The term "vegetative" describes only the medical condition; to refer to a person as a "vegetable" demeans him and his human dignity. Persons in such states are at the mercy of their caregivers, which does not diminish their value as human beings. We should care for them according to their dignity as human persons and children of God until their natural death, providing pain relief, nutrition, hydration, hygiene, warmth, and human affection and preventing complications related to bed confinement.

Rational Limits to Medical Treatment

The medical treatment for a patient in danger of dying can be ethically (as opposed to medically) ordinary or extraordinary in terms of the expected outcome for that patient. Ethically *ordinary* treatment is not excessively burdensome, but is proportionate in its burdens to the foreseeable results for the patient. Ordinary treatment normally includes common health care prescribed to meet real patient needs, such as the use of most pharmaceuticals (antibiotics, anti-inflammatories, blood pressure medication) and many types of surgery.

A treatment is ethically *extraordinary* if it is extremely risky or expensive, if it is not readily available in the patient's setting, or if it increases the patient's suffering.[3] Such a treatment is morally optional because its burden—that is, its risk, expense, or associated discomfort—is out of proportion to its expected results.

Ordinary treatment must always be given to a dying patient, but a patient may decline extraordinary means, even if forgoing such treatment means indirectly hastening death.[4]

The dividing line between ethically ordinary and extraordinary treatments is not rigid. A heart-valve operation may be economically burdensome for one patient, for example, but might constitute ordinary care for another. Use of a mechanical respirator would be *ordinary* for a young person experiencing temporary breathing paralysis (as in Guillain-Barré syndrome) but *extraordinary* for a patient with lung cancer that has spread throughout the body, since it would not produce a proportionate benefit.

In addition, treatments that were previously considered extraordinary become ordinary when scientific progress reduces their risk—as has happened, for example, with the development of minimally invasive surgical techniques.

Therapeutic Tyranny

It is not necessary to employ every possible treatment to keep a patient alive. Aggressive medical interventions do help patients who are experiencing severe but short-lived trauma, but they may also artificially delay death almost indefinitely without providing any real benefit to a patient. When death is inevitable and imminent, an intervention like cardiopulmonary resuscitation or use of an artificial respirator intensifies suffering unnecessarily, because the patient has little likelihood of recovering normal heart or lung function.

Pope St. John Paul II calls such interventions *therapeutic tyranny*. They artificially prolong the agony of dying and "are by now disproportionate to any expected results or because they impose an excessive burden on the patient and his family."[5] Refusing such ethically extraordinary treatment means that the patient can embrace his human condition in the face of death. Refusal is in no way suicide or euthanasia.

Health Care and Suffering

Life includes suffering: losing a loved-one or experiencing defeat and failure, loneliness, misunderstanding, physical and emotional abuse, and pain. Suffering arises from sin; it exists because evil exists. Christ does not want people to suffer, but He embraced suffering so as to redeem it: "With his stripes we are healed" (Isa. 53:5 KJV; 1 Peter 2:24).

Christ gives meaning to suffering, making it redemptive. By uniting their suffering—whether great or small—to Christ and bearing it patiently, the sick and the dying please God, who sees the suffering of his own Son, Jesus Christ, reflected in them. This helps them save others and themselves. St. Paul says, "In my flesh I complete what is lacking in Christ's afflictions for the sake of his body, that is, the Church" (Col. 1:24).

Despite suffering's benefits, we should always work to alleviate it and to accompany the patient, especially when the hope for a cure diminishes. Palliative care—including the use of analgesics and sedatives to control pain—seeks "to make suffering more bearable in the final stages of illness and to ensure that the patient is supported and accompanied in his or her ordeal."[6]

Palliative care neither prolongs life nor causes death. To provide palliative care is to practice true mercy; it is not to kill an innocent person. Palliative care alleviates patients' suffering and reduces their pain; it means providing comfort and accompanying them as persons, giving them "confidence and hope ... [that] makes them reconciled to death."[7] Frequently, patients want to die simply because they feel abandoned or are not given proper pain relief. Every person deserves respect and care in his suffering, not "elimination."

For years the Catholic Church has encouraged advances in palliative care. When other available medications do not alleviate pain, the Church affirms the morality of using narcotics as long as it does not prevent the patient from fulfilling his religious and moral duties, even though it may limit consciousness and indirectly shorten the patient's life.[8]

Care for a Patient with a Degenerative Disease

Besides facing death itself, a patient with a degenerative illness like Parkinson's or Alzheimer's disease must face a long dying process, a gradual, progressive degeneration that may take years. This often raises "quality-of-life" issues for the patient's last days.

The diagnosis of a degenerative illness can arouse intense emotions, leading some patients to wish for a quick death. Such thoughts do not imply "a true desire for euthanasia" but rather "an anguished plea for help and love," especially for companionship and consolation in their difficulties.[9] We must assure patients that we will never abandon them or consider them a burden, and must show them that we will attend to them with love. We should help them pray, to unite their sufferings to Christ's (Col. 1:24) and to ready themselves to be with God.

"Quality of life" is not a criterion for making moral decisions. Life is good in itself—not because of the comfort, ease, or enjoyment we experience—and should be treated as sacred. Human companionship and good palliative care and symptoms management ensure a fitting end of life, as well as a dignified and peaceful process of facing death. Such care also enables patients to fulfill family obligations and prepare for their definitive encounter with God.

The Moment of Death

Advanced techniques for resuscitation and organ transplantation require a precise diagnosis of the exact moment of death. Backed by honest studies and investigation, it is medicine that must define "in the most precise way possible the exact moment and the irrefutable sign of death," and it is medical professionals who have the responsibility to interpret these signs.[10] Medically, death is the "permanent cessation of all vital functions," classically recognized in the definitive shutdown of heart and lungs. Doctors continue to diagnose and certify death using the traditional cardiopulmonary criteria in most cases.[11]

In recent years, however, the use of life support has meant that in some cases a patient's circulation and respiration can be maintained artificially for an indefinite period. This has led to the development of the neurological criteria for determining death, known as the brain-death criteria. Since the brain integrates and coordinates the body's physical and mental functions, "cerebral death is the true criterion of death, since the definitive arrest of the cardio-respiratory functions leads very quickly to cerebral death."[12]

True brain death consists in "the complete and irreversible cessation of all brain activity (in the cerebrum, cerebellum and brain stem). This is then considered the sign that the individual organism has lost its integrative capacity." [13] As used in this definition, *brain* means the entire nervous system within the cranium as a whole: the cerebrum, the cerebellum, and the brain stem.[14] This definition obliges scientists to rigorously and objectively ascertain when all cerebral, cerebellar, and brain-stem activity has completely and irreversibly stopped. This criterion is completely consistent with Catholic teaching on the dignity of the human person.[15]

Advance Medical Directives (Living Wills)

An advance medical directive, also known as a living will, is a legal document in which a person indicates how he or she wishes to be treated in an urgent or terminal-care situation, specifying in particular which medical procedures he would like to receive or avoid if he becomes incompetent (that is, lacking the power to act). An advance directive may include, for example, do-not-resuscitate instructions in the event of cardiac arrest.

An advance directive should respect moral laws when expressing the patient's will regarding possible treatment. It may identify a proxy decision maker for the final moments of life as well as provide instructions about what the proxy is permitted or not permitted to decide. Unfortunately, many living wills are ambiguous and may thus increase the patient's risk of undergoing useless or improper treatment. Some inadvertently permit doctors to euthanize the very persons they are intended to protect.[16]

There is nothing immoral about an advance directive in itself. Catholics should, however, use reasonable care to guarantee that an advance directive is implemented in accordance with the Catholic faith and teachings about death and the dignity of the dying person. The document should use clear language, avoiding ambiguous wording that might be difficult to interpret. It should insist that the individual be regarded as a human person with dignity right up to his natural end. It should also exclude any form of euthanasia and any irrational extension of the dying process.

An advance directive should require that the patient receive medical treatments proportionate to his medical condition, including palliative relief. It may allow the use of sedatives and analgesics even when these may limit consciousness or indirectly shorten the life span. In all circumstances, including diagnosis of a persistent vegetative state, the document should prohibit neglect or withdrawal of normal care, such as the provision of nutrition, hydration, and warmth. To interrupt feeding or hydration is rarely morally justifiable.

Above all, advance directives should insist on respecting and assisting the patient in fulfilling his moral and religious duties, stating his right and desire to receive the sacraments in a timely fashion and to be accompanied by family members through the process of dying.

Building a Culture of Life

Culture is a way of living and thinking that molds a society and orients it toward a particular way of viewing and relating to nature, people, and God. Culture reflects the soul of a nation and molds its youth. It incorporates our values as well as our social, political, artistic, and religious institutions. Unfortunately, culture can include an orientation toward evil and violence, which is often expressed in hedonistic, consumeristic, and atheistic elements.

Popes John Paul II, Benedict XVI, and Francis encourage a culture of life that cultivates and defends human dignity through all stages of life and recovers the culture's most essential element—that is, man's relationship with God. It respects life from its beginning at conception until its natural end, protecting and encouraging it through social, economic, political, and legal institutions.

Parents contribute to the culture of life by educating their children to see life as a gift from God. Young people can transmit the Gospel of life and love to their friends and companions by not giving in to fear or complacency. All Catholics, in every circumstance, can and must build a culture of life.

Notes

1 John Paul II, *Evangelium vitae* (March 25, 1995), n. 65.

2 "Disability-Rights Activist, Once Considered a 'Vegetable,' Joins Fight for Terri Schiavo," *Catholic News Agency*, March 3, 2005, http://www.catholicnewsagency.com/.

3 See Elio Sgreccia, *Personalist Bioethics: Foundations and Applications*, trans. John Di Camillo and Michael Miller (Philadelphia: National Catholic Bioethics Center, 2012), 685. See also Congregation for the Doctrine of the Faith (CDF), *Declaration on Euthanasia* (May 5, 1980), IV.

4 See Pontifical Council "Cor Unum," *Questions of Ethics regarding the Fatally Ill and the Dying* (June 27, 1981), 2.4.3, http://www.academiavita.org/_pdf/magisterium/councils/pontifical_council_cor_unum/fatally_ill_and_dying.pdf. See also Sgreccia, *Personalist Bioethics*, 683.

5 John Paul II, *Evangelium vitae*, n. 65.

6 Ibid.

7 Pontifical Council for Health Care Workers, *Charter for Health Care Workers* (Vatican City: Libreria Editrice Vaticana, 1995), n. 117. See also Pontifical Council "Cor Unum," *Questions of Ethics*, 4.3.

8 Pius XII, Address on the Religious and Moral Implications of Analgesia (February 24, 1957).

9 CDF, *Declaration on Euthanasia*, II; and Pontifical Council for Health Care Workers, *Charter*, n. 149.

10 Pontifical Council for Health Care Workers, *Charter*, n. 128.

[11] Charles B. Clayman, *American Medical Association Encyclopedia of Medicine* (New York: Random House, 1989).

[12] "The Artificial Prolongation of Life: Report of a Pontifical Academy of Sciences Study Group," *Origins* 15.25 (December 5, 1985): 415; and Carlos Chaga, ed., *Working Group on the Artificial Prolongation of Life and the Determination of the Exact Moment of Death, October 19–21, 1985*, PAS Scripta Varia 60 (Vatican City: Pontifical Academy of Sciences, 1986), 113.

[13] John Paul II, Address to the Eighteenth International Congress of the Transplantation Society (August 29, 2000), n. 5.

[14] Eelco F. M. Wijdicks, "The Diagnosis of Brain Death," *New England Journal of Medicine* 344.16 (April 19, 2001): 1215–1221.

[15] See John Paul II, Address to Transplantation Society, n. 5.

[16] Sgreccia, *Personalist Bioethics*, 704.

GLOSSARY

adult stem cells. Located in bodily tissues and organs and capable of renewing indefinitely, these undifferentiated cells can become whatever specialized cell type is needed to repair or maintain the tissue or organ in which they are located. Also called somatic stem cells, they can be obtained from umbilical cords, placentas, amniotic fluid, and cadavers as well as from the bodies of living children and adults. Unlike *embryonic stem cells*, their use does not require the destruction of a human embryo.

Alphonsus Liguori. St. Alphonsus Maria de Liguori (1696–1786) was a priest who founded the religious order of the Congregation of the Most Holy Redeemer (Redemptorists) in 1732. The Church canonized him in 1839 and in 1871 named him a Doctor of the Church. Alphonsus is the patron saint of moral theologians and confessors. His feast day is August 1.

anovulant. A contraceptive that prevents conception by inhibiting ovulation. The most common anovulants are pills containing either progestin alone (the "mini pill") or a combination of estrogen and progestin (the common birth control pill). Anovulants can also be administered by patch, implant, or injection.

anthropology. The study of the human being in his physical, moral, and spiritual dimensions.

assisted reproductive technology (ART). Procedures in which eggs are surgically removed from a woman's ovaries, combined with sperm, and returned to the body of the egg donor or another woman.

bioethics. Study based on foundational principles for analyzing ethical issues in the fields of biology, medical research and practice, and health care policy.

blastocyst. The early-stage embryo that develops from the zygote after about four or five days. The blastocyst is made up of an inner cell mass, which develops into the baby's body, surrounded by an outer layer of cells, which becomes the placenta. Embryonic stem cells are removed from the inner cell mass, destroying the life of the embryo.

brain death. The cessation of all sensory and cognitive functions in the entire brain, including the brain stem. Pope St. John Paul II says, "A health worker professionally responsible for ascertaining death can use these criteria in each individual case as the basis for arriving at that degree of assurance in ethical judgment which moral teaching describes as 'moral certainty'" (Address to the Eighteenth International Congress of the Transplant Society, August 29, 2000).

cardiopulmonary death. Cessation of heart contractions and absence of heartbeat, which lead to anoxia (lack of oxygen in the blood) and eventually death.

chorionic villi. Small projections from the placental membrane that form part of the border between maternal and fetal blood. The villi contain both maternal and fetal cells.

chromosome. A rod-like structure in the nucleus of a cell that holds the linear array of genes. Every human cell contains twenty-three pairs of chromosomes, one chromosome of each pair from the mother and one from the father.

companionship. A healing gift we give to those who are sick. The Congregation for the Doctrine of the Faith notes that "what a sick person needs, besides medical care, is love, the human and supernatural warmth with which the sick person can and ought to be surrounded by those close to him or her, parents and children, doctors and nurses" (*Declaration on Euthanasia*, 1980).

conception. The formation of an embryo by the union of an ovum and sperm. Conception marks the very beginning of human life.

conclave. The confidential meeting of the college of cardinals to elect a new pope.

cooperation in evil. Assisting a person or organization in performing a morally objectionable act, either by formally sharing in the intention of the act or by providing material support. Cooperation may incur culpability depending on its type and degree. See also *formal cooperation* and *material cooperation*.

cryopreservation. The preservation of cells or tissues by freezing. Thousands of human embryos that were created during in vitro fertilization procedures but not implanted are currently stored by cryopreservation. Proposals to use these embryos for research, to implant them, or to destroy them are all ethically problematic. This leaves the embryos in "a situation of injustice which in fact cannot be resolved" (Congregation for the Doctrine of the Faith, *Dignitas personae*, n. 19).

culture of life. The theological position that human life at all stages from conception through natural death is sacred. The culture-of-life doctrine opposes practices that are harmful to human life, including abortion, euthanasia, the destruction of human embryos, contraception, capital punishment, and unjust war. The expression "culture of life" was first used by Pope St. John Paul II at World Youth Day in Denver, Colorado, in 1993.

death. The separation of the spiritual soul from the material body. Pope St. John Paul II says that death "is a single event, consisting in the total disintegration of that unitary and integrated whole that is the personal self" (Address to the Eighteenth International Congress of the Transplant Society, August 29, 2000). Pope Pius XII notes that "it remains for the doctor, and especially the anesthesiologist, to give a clear and precise definition of 'death' and the 'moment of death' of a patient who passes away in a state of unconsciousness" (Address to an International Congress of Anesthesiologists, November 24, 1957).

dehumanization. A view of the human person that reduces respect for human dignity by negating the person's uniqueness, inviolability, sacredness, free will, or transcendent vocation. One example is the notion that complex human behaviors and disorders can be explained by the presence or absence of genes alone.

disproportionate to expected results. A phrase used to describe medical procedures that are more aggressive than their outcomes warrant. Pope St. John Paul II notes that a patient may "forgo so-called 'aggressive medical treatment,' in other words, medical procedures which no longer correspond to the real situation of the patient" so long as normal care is not interrupted (*Evangelium vitae*, n. 65).

DNA. Deoxyribonucleic acid, the molecule that encodes genetic information in the nucleus of every cell. It is made up of four subunits—adenine, cytosine, guanine, and thymine.

Down syndrome. A common genetic condition caused by the presence of a full or partial third copy of chromosome 21; also known as trisomy 21. Common characteristics of persons with Down syndrome include varying degrees of developmental delays, a distinctive set of facial characteristics, low muscle tone, small stature, and mild to moderate intellectual disability, though each case is unique. Early interventions and education about the disorder can greatly increase the quality of life of persons with Down syndrome.

embryo. The new organism that results when a sperm fertilizes an ovum. The resulting organism possesses half the DNA of each parent. In human beings, a newly conceived life is called an embryo for the first eight weeks.

embryonic stem cells. Undifferentiated cells derived from the destruction of an early embryo (see **blastocyst**). Embryonic stem cells derived from the inner cell mass of the blastocyst are pluripotent and possess the capacity to divide for long periods.

"emergency" contraception. Birth control measures used after intercourse. They include the so-called morning-after pills—levonorgestrel (Plan B One-Step) and ulipristal acetate (Ella)—and intrauterine devices. Evidence points to possible abortifacient effects, meaning that these measures are likely in some cases to prevent implantation rather than conception.

ethics. The branch of philosophy that studies human behavior in terms of moral good and evil, virtue, character, value, and purpose or ends. The word *ethics* derives from the Greek *ethos*, meaning "custom, habitual way of acting, or character."

eugenics. A social movement popularized in the early twentieth century, which attempts to improve the human race by "good breeding," reducing and removing people deemed unfit for life (from the Greek *eu*, good, and *genos*, race). Contemporary eugenics involves manipulating embryos to produce desirable genetic traits and eliminate undesirable ones.

euthanasia. "An act or omission which, of itself or by intention, causes death in order to eliminate suffering." Euthanasia puts an end "to the lives of handicapped, sick, or dying persons. It is morally unacceptable" (*Catechism*, n. 2277).

extraordinary (disproportionate) medical treatments. Treatments that "in the patient's judgment do not offer a reasonable hope of benefit, or entail an excessive burden or impose excessive expense on the family or the community." A patient "may forgo extraordinary or disproportionate means of preserving life" (*ERDs*, n. 57).

formal cooperation in evil. Any physical or moral assistance knowingly given to a morally objectionable act by a person who shares the intention of the evildoer, that is, who agrees with the wrongful action and provides assistance in accomplishing it. Formal cooperation is always blameworthy.

gametes. Mature reproductive cells. Gametes contain a single set of unpaired chromosomes. Female gametes are eggs, or ova, and male gametes are sperm. Gametes are also known as germ cells, reproductive cells, or sex cells.

gamete intrafallopian transfer (GIFT). An assisted reproductive technology in which eggs are removed from a woman's ovaries and placed with sperm in one of her fallopian tubes, allowing fertilization to take place at its usual site inside the fallopian tubes.

gene. The fundamental physical and functional unit of heredity that influences human development, growth, and life. Genes are made of hundreds or thousands of DNA bases.

germ cells. See *gametes.*

genetic engineering (genetic manipulation). The intentional alteration or selection of genetic characteristics of a human person, plant, or animal by the insertion or removal of DNA or genes or by selective reproduction based on genetic analysis.

genetic testing. An analysis of DNA, chromosomes, and gene products for inherited genetic disease, to determine genetic risks for offspring, to guide medical treatment, or to further research and individual identification.

Hippocrates. An ancient Greek physician (c. 460 BC to c. 370 BC) who is considered the father of Western medicine. Hippocrates is commonly portrayed as the paragon of the ancient physician, and is credited with the Hippocratic Oath, which is still in use today.

human being. An organism of the species *Homo sapiens.*

human dignity. A fundamental, inalienable quality possessed by every person. Because they are made in the image of God and destined to share eternally in God's own life, human beings possess a sacred dignity. (See *Catechism*, nn. 355–384, esp. n. 356.) The human person is never to be treated as a thing or as a means to an end.

human genome. The complete set of genes that every person inherits from his or her parents. It is present in virtually every cell of the body.

human papillomavirus (HPV). The most common sexually transmitted virus, which may cause genital warts and cancer. More than forty types of HPV are known.

in vitro fertilization (IVF). An assisted reproductive technology in which eggs and sperm are brought together in a laboratory dish (*in vitro* literally means "in glass") to allow the sperm to fertilize an egg. IVF is performed with any combination of spousal and donor eggs and sperm.

induced pluripotent stem cells (iPSCs). Cells that have been genetically reprogrammed to an embryonic-like undifferentiated stem cell state. Developed from a patient's own cells, these cells do not require the destruction of embryos and can be used to grow therapeutic tissues perfectly matched to the patient. Also called reprogrammed adult stem cells.

live attenuated vaccine. A vaccine produced from a virus whose original virulence has been diminished so that it causes little or no disease. The attenuated virus reproduces slowly in the vaccinated individual and elicits an excellent immune response.

luteinizing hormone. A hormone that occurs naturally during a woman's cycle, which triggers ovulation and the development of the corpus luteum.

magisterium. The authentic teaching office of the Church, which consists of the Pope and the bishops in union with him.

material cooperation in evil. Physical or moral assistance knowingly given to a morally objectionable act by a person who does not share the same intention as the evildoer but nonetheless contributes to the act for another reason. Material cooperation may or may not be blameworthy, depending on how close the cooperation is to the action.

natural law. "The original moral sense which enables man to discern by reason the good and the evil, the truth and the lie" (*Catechism*, n. 1954). Natural law is common to all humanity, knowable by all through reason, and objectively true. The first precept of natural law, according to St. Thomas Aquinas (1225–1274), is that "good is to be done and evil is to be avoided" (*Summa theologiae* I-II.94.2).

ordinary (proportionate) medical treatments. Treatments that "in the judgment of the patient offer a reasonable hope of benefit and do not entail an excessive burden or impose excessive expense on the family or the community." A patient "has a moral obligation to use ordinary or proportionate means of preserving his or her life" (*ERDs*, n. 56).

ovarian hyperstimulation syndrome. A condition in which the ovaries become swollen and painful, resulting from the injection of a hormone called human chorionic gonadotropin (hCG) to induce the release of eggs. In severe cases, OHSS includes rapid weight gain, abdominal pain, vomiting, and shortness of breath. Oral fertility drugs such as clomiphene can also cause OHSS, though this is rarer.

passive cooperation in evil. Moral assistance knowingly given to a morally objectionable act by a person who does not denounce or impede the act when it is carried out by another person.

persistent vegetative state (PVS). A coma-like state that occurs when a patient can only perform certain involuntary actions on his or her own and exhibits no reproducible voluntary responses to external stimuli. A patient in a PVS lacks language expression and seems to lack comprehension, though this remains controversial. The lower brain stem in PVS patients is still healthy and fully functioning.

personalist norm. Pope St. John Paul II writes that the "personalist norm, in its negative aspect, states that the person is the kind of good which does not admit of use and cannot be treated as an object of use and as the means to an end. In its positive form the personalist norm says that the person is a good toward which the only proper and adequate attitude is love" (*Love and Responsibility*, Ignatius, 41).

pluripotency. The capacity of certain stem cells to develop into any specialized cell type in the body, including nerve cells, heart cells, bone cells, and skin cells. Embryonic stem cells (obtained by fetal destruction) and iPSCs (which do not involve fetal destruction) are both pluripotent.

preimplantation genetic diagnosis (PGD). A laboratory technique used to screen embryos for genetic defects by removing one or two cells at the six- to ten-cell stage. Embryos with genetic problems are destroyed, while those free of problematic genes are placed in the uterus or frozen for future use.

prenatal genetic testing. Testing of a fetus before birth to detect genetic disorders.

savior sibling. A child conceived through IVF and selected for implantation using preimplantation genetic diagnosis, whose cord blood, bodily cells, tissues, or organs are intended to provide therapy for an older sibling affected with a fatal disease, such as cancer or certain forms of anemia.

zygote. The first stage of human life, which begins with the single cell that forms when an ovum and a sperm cell merge. In human beings, the zygote travels down the fallopian tube and divides rapidly. After about five days, the cells develop into an inner fluid-filled cavity and become a blastocyst, which then embeds in the endometrial lining of the uterus.